Safe, Scenic, and

Traffic-Free Bicycling

A Fireside Book

Published by Simon & Schuster

New York London Toronto Sydney Tokyo Singapore

The Best

Bike Paths of

the Southwest

Wendy Williams

For Carl and Danny Bair,

my Arizona guides.

Thanks.

F

FIRESIDE
Rockefeller Center
1230 Avenue of the Americas
New York, NY 10020

FIRESIDE and colophon are registered trademarks
of Simon & Schuster, Inc.

DESIGNED BY BARBARA MARKS
MAPS BY DANIEL CHIU

Manufactured in the United States of America

10 9 8 7 6 5 4 3 2 1

Library of Congress Cataloging-in-Publication Data
Williams, Wendy, date
    The best bike paths of the Southwest : safe, scenic, and traffic-free
    bicycling / Wendy Williams.
        p.   cm.
    "A Fireside book."
    1. Bicycle touring—Southwest, New—Guidebooks.   2. Bicycle
trails—Southwest, New—Guidebooks.   3. Southwest, New—Guidebooks.
I. Title.
GV1045.5.S678W45   1996
796.6'4'0979—dc20   95-26747
                                                        CIP

ISBN 0-684-81400-5

Contents

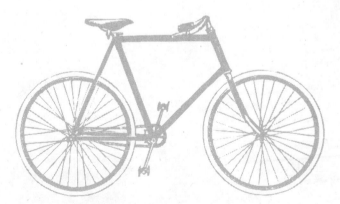

Introduction

I
n Northern California, you can ride along the American River for 32.8 miles and worry more about seeing a mountain lion than about meeting a high-speed semi. Along the Sacramento River, you can pedal past boarded-up gold mines and cross the river on one of the nation's most beautiful bikes-only bridges.

In Yosemite you can leave your car and pedal through the valley on a bike path that takes you to that park's most popular places. In Southern California, you can see San Diego and the elegance of the resort city of Coronado, all from the oceanside paved path.

Arizona has rides through magical saguaro forests, and Utah has riverside and canyon rides that lead to waterfalls and state parks. All across America, miles of these exquisite paved paths are being built each month. This burgeoning network is creating a new form of biking, bringing "accessible adventure" to families, enabling parents with young children or older adults to plan safe and scenic bike rides through some of America's most beautiful settings.

But where are they? America's paved-path network is a grass-roots system, built bit by bit, as various groups and people have become involved. Sponsoring organizations have included the federal Department of Transportation, the National Park Service, state transportation departments and state parks, small municipalities, community activist groups, and even, in a few cases, private organizations funded by individual donations.

Because of this diversity, a comprehensive listing and description of America's paved paths simply didn't exist. In this book, we've provided the information you'll need to find these hidden treasures. Whether you're a parent planning an outing with young children, an avid cyclist who thinks a 50-mile ride is a short day's work, or an older adult (like me) back in the saddle after a long hiatus, you'll be able to read this book and pick out the rides best suited to you and your cycling companions.

How to Use This Book:

At the beginning of each listing, we've included a few facts to let you know quickly the basic parameters of that particular path: a descriptive sentence that usually includes the one-way length of the path, the level of difficulty, the type of scenery you'll be riding through, and the condition of the path.

We realize that "level of difficulty" is a matter of personal opinion. The descriptions we've used—"easy," "average," "challenging"—are based on our experiences of us: a group of friends, mostly in their mid-40s, who ride once or twice a week on a casual basis. If you are a distance cyclist, you may find some of our "challenging" rides to be rather easy; if you are a parent with a 5-year-old, you may find our "average" rides too difficult. Scale up or down, according to your own abilities and interests.

At the end of each entry, we've listed a contact address and telephone number. Many paths in this book are in transition right now, being lengthened or rebuilt or otherwise improved. For the most up-to-date information, we suggest you contact the listed agency. Sometimes these agencies can also help you with other questions, including where to stay or what other activities might be available.

Rules of the Road and Other Necessities:

Most states now have laws requiring children to wear helmets when cycling. We suggest that helmets are appropriate for everyone.

Also good to bring: plenty of water, a quick-energy snack, a tire-patch kit, a first-aid kit, and a bike lock.

In general, bike and recreation paths are like automobile roads. The rules are pretty much the same. Usually everyone is asked to keep to the right; to signal when passing; to maintain reasonable speed limits; and to respect the rights of others. If you are riding with friends, don't ride abreast, blocking the way for others. If you stop to rest, pull off the path onto the shoulder. Some of the newer paths even have scenic rest areas, attractive places with benches or picnic tables where you can talk, eat, or make repairs without impeding traffic.

Recreation paths are not appropriate places for high-speed cycling. They are for recreation and welcome anyone, from children on tricycles to seniors out for a stroll. Acceptable speeds range from about 5 miles per hour to about 20 miles per hour.

A Word to In-Line Skaters:

In-line skaters and cyclists coexist comfortably on today's wide recreation paths; most paths in this book welcome in-line skaters and walkers as well as cyclists. In the few places where we have seen skating expressly forbidden, we have mentioned it. However, this can change. If you want to skate on a particular path, we suggest you check ahead to be sure.

Keep in mind that recreation paths are *not* appropriate places to teach young children how to skate or cycle; we've seen serious accidents result when tottering children fell in front of oncoming cyclists.

In California, where we saw some astonishingly facile in-line skaters, cyclists and skaters mixed happily, making room for each other's styles with gracious acceptance. All it takes is mutual tolerance. The cyclists respected the skaters' need for extra sideways maneuverability, while the skaters moved over quickly when faster cyclists called out politely from behind.

The Best
Bike Paths of
the Southwest

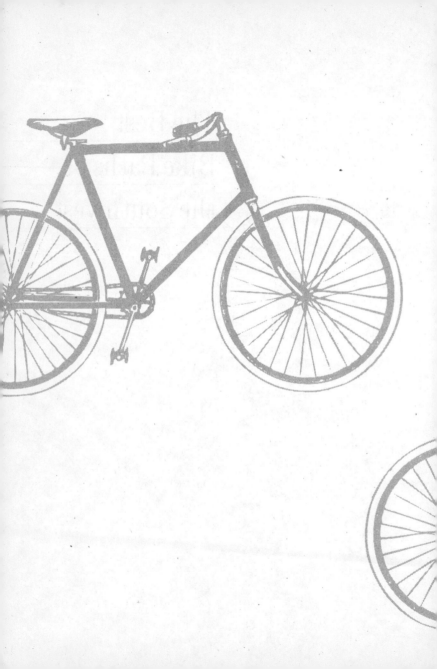

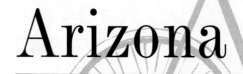

Arizona

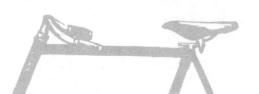

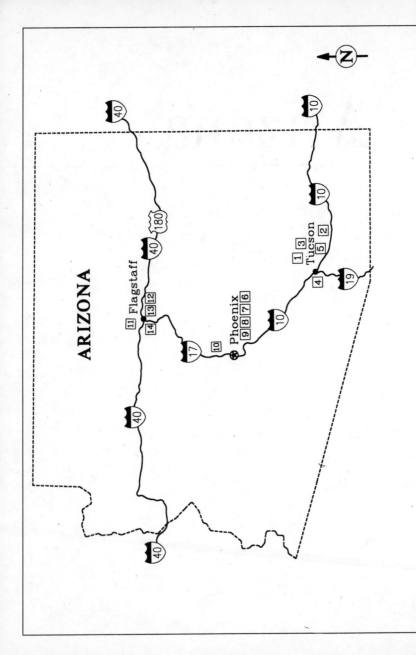

Arizona

1. Sabino Canyon

General Description:

A 3.7-mile narrow canyon road, closed to automobiles, climbing 600 feet through riparian wilderness and dense saguaro cactus forests, crossing and recrossing a freshwater stream on stone bridges built in the 1930s by Emergency Relief employees.

A "best ride"—well worth traveling for!

Level of Difficulty: Very challenging—especially the final 0.7-mile segment through the Upper Canyon.

Type of Scenery: One of the most biologically diverse plant communities in the United States grows on the southeastern canyon wall; the only dependable freshwater stream in the Tucson basin; fantastic riparian ecosystem featuring cool stands of graceful cottonwoods, white-barked Arizona sycamore, and velvet ash with leaves that turn brilliant gold in the brisk fall air; Sonoran mud turtles lurking near the rushing stream and threatened Gila chub swimming in the shallow ponds; evening visits from deer, coyote, and fox; mountain lions and bighorn sheep have been reported.

Condition of Pavement: Good.

General Background:

There are those who say our feeling for natural beauty

is based on our genes, that our love of green hills and flowing water evolved from our survival instincts. They say we *desire* to find, in outdoor life, what our simian ancestors *had* to find—a tall tree for a good night's sleep, cool running water, and some open highland to give a clear view of whatever might be lurking out there.

If so, it's easy to imagine our simian ancestors being drawn to the safety and security of Sabino Canyon and then coming to love its beauty. The canyon's creek, the only dependable freshwater in the Tucson Basin, flows out of the 9,000-foot-high Santa Catalina Mountains, a range of rickety peaks that tend to fall apart and slide into each other from time to time.

The creek first began to flow after the peaks were formed, over a 7-million-year period, between 12 million and 5 million years ago. Over the eons, the water gnashed at the canyon rock, chewing it into sand and pebbles that were carried off in the floodwaters.

Periodically, earthquakes and other geologic cataclysms contributed to the canyon-making. In his book *Sabino Canyon* David Lazaroff describes the people of Tucson watching a mountain peak tumble off its perch and fall into Sabino Canyon. It was on a Tuesday, May 3, 1887. An earthquake centered in Mexico rippled through the dry Southwest. Lazaroff reprinted the *Arizona Daily Star*'s account: "great slices of the mountain gave way. . . . little mountains, wrested from their seats by the shock, came thundering down into the valley."

Neither has Sabino Canyon always been a desert. There was a time when the canyon was tropical. During the Pleistocene period, when ice sheets ebbed and flowed over the continent like ocean water lapping at a flat shore-line, Sabino was sometimes wet and cool. About 12,000 years ago, the canyon's climate resembled that of today's Northern California, as evidenced by fossilized Douglas fir, ponderosa pine, piñon, juniper, and oak found in 12,000-year-old pack-rat dens.

But hotter temperatures forced the temperate plants to withdraw. The Sonoran Desert plants arrived in waves, like an invading army. A phalanx of saguaro cacti, the desert giants, arrived 8,000 years ago. Next came more sophisticated plants like the palo verdes, trees with chloro-phyll-filled green bark.

Today you'll see long-armed saguaro limb-to-limb with water-dependent cottonwood and sycamore. Canyon ferns live near barrel cactus. Crayfish and snails and endangered fish thrive in the water while only a few feet away subspecies of cholla cactus bake in the sun.

This is the "edge effect," the reason why life thrives in riparian zones and why Sabino Canyon has special biologi-cal importance. Animals living here get two (or three or four) habitats for the price of one admission to the canyon floor. They can sleep and homestead in one zone, travel a few feet to drink in a second zone, and travel only a few feet more to hunt in a third habitat.

Sabino Canyon was almost lost to development, but plans for a dam were delayed by the depression of the 1930s. The federal government built the narrow road up the canyon, but the local citizenry were unable to raise the funds to complete the project.

In the 1970s, the U.S. Forest Service decided the depression-era road was too narrow to accommodate automobile traffic. Today visitors may walk or bike or ride horses up the canyon, or ride the public shuttle ($5 round-trip) to any (or all) of the nine stops along the road.

During the 1970s, cyclists were allowed unlimited use of the canyon road, but there were too many accidents. Cyclists zoomed down the narrow road and around the sharp bends at 40 or 50 miles per hour, frightening walkers and running into oncoming shuttles. Today, cyclists using the road have strictly limited hours (see Special Precautions), must carry identification, and may get speeding tickets.

The Bike Path:

No bikes are allowed in the canyon from 9 A.M. to 5 P.M. You may ride early in the morning, in the evening, or even during the night if you have a bike light. (The canyon never "closes.") During the summer, lots of cyclists ride up after five, picnic and swim, and come back down as late as one or two or three in the morning. There are plenty of places where you can lock your bike and find a solitary place to sit and talk quietly, read, or just meditate.

From the visitor center, the climb starts very gradually. In fact, the first mile actually dips a bit before climbing the canyon. Along this first section, several paved roads branch to the right. To add distance to your ride, you might explore these. If you're not sure you will have the energy for the final Upper Canyon climb (don't underestimate this final difficulty), forget the side trip. Getting to the top of the canyon is more rewarding.

After the easy first mile, you'll enter the canyon itself. Hemmed in by the steep canyon walls, you'll start climbing. You won't *see* Sabino Creek at first. You'll *hear* it. It's the friendly sound, the steady base note under the treble of birdsong and windsong echoing off the surrounding walls.

When the road bends sharply east, the creek appears at last. The rushing water, the saguaro-covered canyon walls, the narrow depression-era stone bridges shaded by leafy trees—this is the canyon at its most hypnotizing. For the next mile or so, any time you want to you can stop and wade in the water or rest by the shallow, rock-lined pools.

Continuing along the road, you'll eventually climb above the flowing water, riding high up into the ever-narrowing canyon. You may see hikers above you on a narrow ridge trail. If the cliffs themselves seem familiar, this isn't déjà vu. Lots of chase-the-outlaw Westerns have been filmed here.

The last 0.7-mile will challenge any cyclist. Do try to get to the top—there are some great things to see. Lock your bike and walk up if you're too tired to ride. At the end of the paved road, you can lock your bike and hike about a half-mile up the Phone Line Trail (there are three switch-backs), where there are great views of the basin.

Food Facilities Nearby: None.

Restrooms: At the visitor center; non-flush toilets at frequent stops along the canyon road.

Special Precautions: There are strict rules for cyclists who ride here. This is to prevent the serious cycling accidents that have occurred in past years. Here are a few of the rules. For a complete list, contact the address below.

- *No* bicycling allowed on Wednesdays and Saturdays.
- The road is closed to bikes every day from 9 A.M. to 5 P.M.
- The *strict* speed limit is 15 miles per hour.
- All cyclists over the age of 14 must carry identification with a photograph. Failure to provide an ID may result in confiscation of the cyclist's front wheel!
- Only four cyclists per group.
- There are more "safety mitigation measures," designed to protect cyclists *and* pedestrians.

In addition, Forest Service officials warn about thunderstorms. People have been killed by lightning in this canyon.

Water running over the road and bridges can be dangerous.

Snakes warm themselves in the evening by stretching across the canyon road. Beware!

Bring *plenty* of drinking water.

Best Parking Lot: The Sabino Canyon Visitor Center.

Directions: From I-10, take the Grand Road exit and head east. Go 6 miles. Turn left (north) on Swan. Go 4.1 miles. Turn right (east) on Sunrise. Go 4.2 miles. At the "**T**," you will have reached Sabino Canyon Road. Turn left. Parking is immediately on your right.

For More Information: Sabino Canyon Visitor Center, the Coronado National Forest of the U.S. Forest Service, 5700 North Sabino Canyon Road, Tucson, Arizona 85715. Tel.: (520) 749-8700.

2. The Old Spanish Trail and the Cactus Forest Loop Drive of the Saguaro National Park (East)

General Description:

A 5.8-mile path paralleling a busy but pretty road through the foothills of the Rincon Mountains; and an 8.3-mile loop through the national park, along a narrow road that allows cars, but at speeds no greater than 25 miles per hour.

Level of Difficulty: Challenging.

Type of Scenery: The Rincon Mountains east of Tucson; rolling climbs and descents with views of the Santa Catalina Mountains to the north, the Tucson Mountains to the west, and the city of Tucson below; homes and buildings, but not congested; the desert hills inside Saguaro National Park (East).

Condition of Pavement: Good, but with some potholes.

General Background:

The beauty of the desert is a beauty of texture, a beauty of distance and height and intensity of contrast. In this world, the harsh saguaro cactus is startling.

Were you to describe a saguaro to someone who'd never seen one, your words—"tall, prickly, and medium to light green with many protuberances"—would fail dismally to express the stunning presence of this plant. Arizona's giant saguaro is as majestic as California's giant redwood, and just as unique. Nowhere else but in the Sonoran Desert will you find a cactus that's 50 feet high, weighs 8 tons, and gesticulates to the world with 7 or 8 withered old arms.

Saguaros are quite delicate when young. A saguaro produces about 40 million seeds in its lifetime, but very few seedlings survive. Some seeds are eaten by animals, and some are destroyed by frosts. They grow excruciatingly slowly. First-year seedlings stand ¼ inch high; 15-year-olds reach 1 foot; and 50-year-olds, about 7 feet. They don't sprout limbs (and some saguaros never sprout them) until after they have flowered for the first time, at about 50 years old. When you see a 50-foot-tall, many-limbed saguaro, you're looking at something born at about the time America was born, 200 years ago.

In Saguaro National Park, you'll get a change to see some of the oldest saguaros in the Sonoran Desert. These slopes seem to have the optimum amount of cold and heat, the optimum amount of rain and sun, so that the cacti thrive here better than anywhere else. The park's area has been protected since 1933; cattle grazing has been eliminated and vandalism curtailed, somewhat.

You'll see some other good examples of Sonoran Desert vegetation, too, including fields of wildflowers like deep purple lupines and bright red beardtongue penstemon, if you're lucky enough to ride through during the spring.

The Bike Path:

The Old Spanish Trail bike path parallels an automobile road of the same name from Tucson to the national park. Cyclists ride out on Old Spanish Trail from Tucson, loop around the national park road, and return to the city along the same bike path, a challenging ride of about 20 miles. You should be physically fit and accustomed to desert heat.

The Spanish Trail bike path begins in Tucson at the intersection of two roads: Old Spanish Trail and Broadway. The path's first 3 miles resemble a sidewalk so much that many cyclists prefer the striped bike lane on the automobile road.

When you cross Houghton Road, the bike path improves. Cyclists who prefer a shorter ride might begin from here, rather than from Broadway. After the intersection of Houghton Road and Old Spanish Trail, the hills become long and rolling and the views become more open. You'll see lots of distance here, including miles of open rangeland. The large apartment complexes disappear; development (for now, anyway) is rather sparse.

The bike path begins climbing at this point, so that you'll be riding up a mild but persistent grade until you reach the national park. The path curves and bends interestingly. You're riding a 300-year-old trail followed by Spanish soldiers and explorers. The undulation is a welcome relief from Arizona's monotonously straight highways, but it is challenging.

The Saguaro National Park (East) Visitor Center has a bicycle rest area with water, shade, restrooms, and bike racks, which you are invited to use, even if you don't ride in the park.

The Loop Road:

If you choose to ride there, we promise it will be one of the best rides of your life. But you should be aware of several points.

(1) This *is* an automobile road. A steady stream of cars uses this road every day. Unless you come very early, you can't avoid them. The speed limit is 25 miles per hour. However, most people, here to see the sights, drive slower than that.

(2) This is a one-way loop. Cyclists must ride in the direction of traffic. If you begin the ride and decide it's too difficult, you're out of luck. You *cannot* turn around. You *must* continue in the direction of traffic flow.

(3) This is a hilly, hot, and shadeless road. Don't try it if you aren't in condition. If you get overheated, stop and relax. Walk your bike. Drink some water. There's no hurry.

From Old Spanish Trail, ride in the front gate, past the visitor center and over to the loop road gate. (You'll have to pay $2 per cyclist.) You'll head to the left, along with the traffic flow. Several miles into the loop, a side road veers left to a viewing area. We didn't find this mile-long road any more spectacular than the main road. Unless you have energy to spare, skip it.

For a change of pace, walk along the Desert Ecology Trail that branches off the loop road. This is a 0.25-mile guided walk that emphasizes desert-environment and water-resource issues.

Continuing along the loop road, you'll see the Cactus Forest Trail on your right. This dirt trail cuts the paved loop in half and is the only dirt trail open to bikes. It's a rough ride; only experienced backcountry cyclists should try it.

About 5 miles around the loop, you'll begin a mile-long climb up a ridge. On the slopes just below, you'll see a varied carpet of desert scrub. If you're riding in March or April, you'll see fields of wildflowers, stretches of yellow and blue and red coloring the hillsides.

At the climb's crest, you'll round a bend to see the Tucson Basin and its surrounding mountain ranges. To the north are the Santa Catalinas, where Sabino Canyon (see separate entry) lies. To the west are the Tucson Mountains with their recognizable volcanic shapes. To the distant south are the Santa Rita Mountains. Below this circle of cool peaks, down in the basin, sits the city that sizzles in the desert sun.

The remaining ride is downhill but be aware: the last section of road is two-way and cars will move faster.

Distances:
Along Old Spanish Trail:

From Broadway to Harrison:	1.7 miles
From Harrison to Houghton:	1.3 miles
From Houghton to Saguaro National Park (East):	2.8 miles

Food Facilities Nearby: None.

Restrooms: At the national park visitor center.

Special Precautions: No water is available on Old Spanish Trail or along the 8-mile loop road. There *is* drinking water at the visitor center.

The Spanish Trail bike path is narrow, with sharp bends that may keep you from seeing cyclists coming in the opposite direction.

The loop road allows cars and trucks. The last segment of this loop is two-way; traffic may be moving at 30 or 40 miles per hour (although the speed limit is 25 miles per hour). Keep to your own side!

For the Avid Cyclist: A striped bike lane—*not* a path—continues along the Old Spanish Trail highway from the national park to Colossal Cave, a state park about 10 miles to the southeast.

Best Parking Lot: The visitor center at Saguaro National Park (East); Houghton Road; Broadway. (Parking is catch-as-catch-can along these two roads.)

Directions: To the national park: From I-10 take the Houghton Road exit; go north. Turn right (east) onto Escalante Road. This will take you to the Old Spanish Trail and the national park.

If you continue north along Houghton Road, you will intersect the Old Spanish Trail road and bike path.

To the beginning of the Old Spanish Trail: From I-10, take the Broadway exit and head east. Go east all the way through Tucson, to its eastern edge, more than 9 miles. Cross Pantano Road. Look for the Old Spanish Trail on your right.

For More Information: Alternate Modes Coordinator, City of Tucson, Department of Transportation, P.O. Box 27210, Tucson, Arizona 85726-7210. Tel.: (520) 791-4372.

Saguaro National Park (East), 3693 South Old Spanish Trail, Tucson, Arizona 85730. Tel.: (520) 733-5153.

3. The Rillito River Park Bike Path

General Description:

A 4.5-mile path running along the north bank of a usually dry riverbed, through a series of urban parks emphasizing the water-preservation concepts of "xeriscape" landscaping.

Level of Difficulty: Very easy.
Type of Scenery: Xeriscape landscaping, native desert plantings.
Condition of Pavement: Excellent.

General Background:

Nature's web of complexity is more obvious in the desert than in other environs. In gentler climates, the tenuousness of life, the essentiality of water, and the erosive force of its powerful flow are hidden by lush foliage, fertile soil, and languid brooks.

But in the desert, there is no camouflage. You see life as it really is: tough and violent. The organism that survives does so by scraping its vitality out of bare stone and dry sand.

There is a beauty in this ruggedness, an attractiveness sometimes hard for human eyes to appreciate. The world that appears barren and simple on the surface turns out to be complex, interesting, and alluring on the deeper levels.

This philosophy—that beauty is sometimes comprised of juxtapositions of the simple and the complex—has been applied to modern desert landscaping in a newly developed style called "xeriscape." Xeriscape thrives on variety, even while emphasizing water conservation and the use of plants native to the region.

One of the best places in Arizona to get a look at xeriscape in action is the Rillito River Park Bike Path. During most of this 4.5-mile ride, you'll see a desert world that is, in its own way, lush beyond belief.

If you're riding at the right time of year (March through May), you'll see acres of desert wildflowers laid out before you: fields of yellow desert marigold and Mexican gold poppy, tall stems of deep-purple lupine and blood-red penstemon, bunches of desert bluebells, and spreads of desert globe mallow in pink, red, magenta, and orange.

For height, you'll see acacia trees covered with yellow flowers and palo verdes that survive through the hot summer months, when they may drop their tiny leaves to conserve water, by photosynthesizing with their soft-green chlorophyll-filled bark. For shade, you'll have the desert willow and the mesquite tree.

The color, variety, and texture might surprise you: there's more to the desert than rocks and cacti. But what will startle you most is that these plants *belong* here. Almost everything planted along this path is native to the Southwest, perfectly suited to fit into the desert in a splashy sort of way—but without taking more from the desert than the desert is prepared to give.

The Bike Path:

The bike path begins at Campbell Avenue, on the north side of the bridge over the riverbed. Begin riding to the west and you'll soon pass the Rillito Downs Race Track and Rillito Park, a separate park that connects to the Rillito *River* Park. If you're riding here in the late winter or early spring, during the early morning hours you'll see horses in training, preparing for the afternoon races.

Across from the racetrack, on the other side of the riverbed, is Tucson Mall, the region's largest shopping area. Next door is the Tohono Tadai Transit Center, a brightly colored depot where cyclists can catch a bus and either leave their bikes in bike lockers or take them along: every bus in this city carries a bike rack in front, available for free. You just hitch up your bike and climb on board.

Continuing along the River Park bike path, between Oracle and Flowing Wells Roads you'll find the Children's Memorial Park, a neighborhood park with a memorial wall dedicated to children who have died before reaching adulthood.

Almost at the path's west end, at the confluence of Roller Coaster Wash and the Rillito River, you'll find a most remarkable symbol of the commitment of the people of Tucson to their artists and to their cultural history—a sun circle, reminiscent of Stonehenge, based on the culture of the Anasazi and Tohono O'odham people. A thousand years ago, these cultures used sun circles to keep track of crop periods and ritual days. Sunlight falls in particular places within the sun circle on four special days of the year: summer and winter solstice, and spring and fall equinox. Artists Chris Tanz and Paul Edwards created this

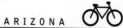

sun circle as part of a Pima County public art program: throughout this county, all public construction projects must spend 1 percent of their budget on public art.

This bike path is unusual in that there are no road crossings, nor are there any sections that run alongside automobile roads. When the bike path crosses any roads, there are underpasses. Each of these underpasses costs several hundred thousand dollars, yet another sign of the commitment of Tucsonans to the development of a world-class biking system.

Food Facilities Nearby: None.
Restrooms: Rillito Park; Children's Memorial Park.
Special Precautions: None.
Best Parking Lot: Rillito Park.
Directions: From I-10, take the Grand Road exit and head east to First Avenue. Turn left on First Avenue and go north, crossing the Rillito River. You'll see a large sign for Rillito Park and large blue monument walls marking the entry.
For More Information: Alternative Modes Coordinator, City of Tucson, Department of Transportation, P.O. Box 27210, Tucson, Arizona 85726-7210. Tel.: (520) 791-4372.

4. The Santa Cruz River Park

General Description:

Two parallel 3.5-mile paths following the east and the west banks of the Santa Cruz River, from Grant Road to Silverlake Road.

Level of Difficulty: Easy.

Type of Scenery: Several nice city parks; lots of city art, areas emphasizing desert landscaping and native plants like velvet mesquite and Fremont cottonwood.

Condition of Pavement: Excellent.

General Background:

City and county bikeway planners intend, within the next several years, to complete the construction of a loop of bike paths running through Tucson. The Santa Cruz path is one of four that will make up this almost contiguous bike-path system. The other three are the Rillito River path (nearly completed); the 4.5-mile Golf Links Bike Path (under construction); and Pantano Wash path (in the dream stage).

When the loop is completed, you'll be able to ride through the city on more than 10 miles of bike paths. The loop will run up the west side of Tucson on the Santa Cruz path, cross the Rillito riverbed on a soon-to-be-built bike bridge, and run down the Rillito bike path to the Pantano

35

Wash. The Pantano Wash path, when complete, will run southeast, to the Old Spanish Trail bike path and the Golf Links bike path that traverses the northern boundary of the Davis-Monthan Air Force Base.

The Bike Path:

Running from north to south near Interstate 10, these two parallel paths follow the east and the west banks of the Santa Cruz River corridor. On the west bank, the path is contiguous; underpasses allow you to avoid busy automobile road crossings. On the east bank, there is no underpass to help cyclists cross Congress Street, a major road. Cyclists must either walk across the Congress Street bridge to the west-bank path or take their chances trying to cross Congress Street on their own. Bike facilities officials prefer that cyclists walk their bikes over the bridge.

The west-bank path is the newer path. Much of the 3.5 miles on this side of the river are dotted with "pocket parks," small and often nameless neighborhood parks that provide intermittent green spaces throughout the urban environment. We particularly liked the mosaics at the pocket park near the St. Mary's Road entrance to the bike path. Tucson always devotes a small portion of construction funds to public art; in this case, $77,000. Five 8-foot-tall pillars stand in this park, covered with brightly colored tiles, hand-painted by artist Susan Gamble. On each pillar the tiles spell out the history of the Santa Cruz River Valley in letters and symbols. Three different languages—English, Spanish, Yaqui—symbolize three of the important cultures that have flourished in the region.

Also on the west bank, running from Mission Lane to

Congress Street, is an interpretive outdoor nature center that features an "acequia," a replica of the irrigation system used by the ancient Hohokam people who lived here before the Europeans arrived. Along the "acequia" you'll find many of the native riparian plants that thrived here during those earlier centuries.

Food Facilities Nearby: None.

Restrooms: At the neighborhood park.

Special Precautions: This is a city path. Ride here with a friend, and only during daylight hours.

Best Parking Lot: At the neighborhood park located between Speedway and St. Mary's Road.

Directions: The park is between Speedway Boulevard and St. Mary's Road. Take the Speedway exit from I-10 and go west. Turn left after the bridge and look for the park.

For More Information: Alternative Modes Coordinator, City of Tucson, Department of Transportation, P.O. Box 27210, Tucson, Arizona 85726-7210. Tel.: (520) 791-4372.

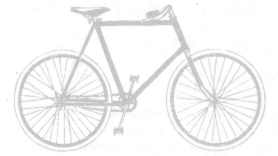

ARIZONA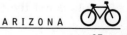

5. The Mountain Avenue Bikeway

General Description:

A 3.5-mile bike-path/bike-lane hybrid, that will link the Rillito River Park Bike Path with the center of Tucson and the University of Arizona, by 1997.

Level of Difficulty: Easy. Caution: This is a bike path/bike lane *hybrid* (see below).

Type of Scenery: Very urban, with lots of public art and desert landscaping; the University of Arizona campus; residential homes with horses standing in many front yards; some fields and pastureland; a large bike-and-pedestrian bridge over the Rillito River, connecting Mountain Avenue with the Rillito River Park Bike Path (see separate entry).

Condition of Pavement: Excellent.

General Background:

This is a "must-ride" for anyone interested in learning how much can be done to encourage safe and pleasant bicycling in the midst of a very busy city environment!

On any day of the week, at just about any daylight hour, you can stand at Mountain Avenue and Grant Road to count the cyclists whizzing along this state-of-the-art bikeway. In less than an hour you'll top 100 riders. Cyclists have always used this main thoroughfare, which runs through the city to the University of Arizona campus, but the newly designed bike thoroughfare has increased use by 30 percent.

That figure is bound to grow when this model project is completed in 1997. Then you'll be able to ride safely and comfortably from Tucson's center all the way to the Rillito River Park Bike Path by way of a 16-foot-wide bike-and-pedestrian bridge that will cost $1 million to build. Ultimately, the Mountain Avenue project will cost $5 million. Tucsonans have made a major financial commitment to city cycling. In doing so, they've created an *attractive* cycling facility that people *want* to use.

The bike path/bike lane hybrid looks like this: On each side of Mountain Avenue is a 16-foot-wide bike-and-pedestrian corridor. Designers didn't want to widen the existing roadway right-of-way; instead, they took footage from the vehicular traffic lanes, reducing them to 11 feet. The plan's designers say this sends a subtle message to motorists about the importance of bikes as transportation.

Included in the bike-and-pedestrian corridors are 3-foot-wide, peach-colored, brick-surfaced buffer zones marking a no-man's-land between motor lane and bike lane. The roadway has been resurfaced with rubberized asphalt, darker than typical asphalt and more likely to hold that color under the heat of the desert sun. Made with recycled automobile tires, rubberized asphalt also lasts longer. The bike lane, on the other hand, is made of gray concrete; there's no mistaking the different purposes of these two lanes,

Designers have included a number of other thoughtful additions. The 5-foot-wide sidewalks are laid out with sculptures and artwork. Public transportation shuttle-stops also have drinking fountains. Trees planted between the sidewalk and the bike lane provide shade. Low-pressure sodium lighting reduces uplighting. (Several astronomical observatories sit on nearby peaks.)

The Bike Path:

Mountain Avenue is a straight road heading north to the Rillito River from the University of Arizona. The bike facility begins at the intersection of Mountain Avenue and 2nd Street, on the university's north side. You'll ride for the first mile on the most extensively developed section. Here, the city has even designed pull-off areas for the shuttle buses, so cyclists don't have to ride out into traffic to get around the stopped buses.

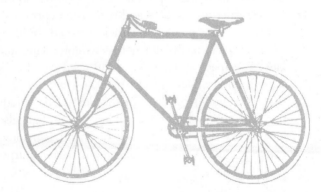

After the first mile, you'll leave the intense urban environment to ride past houses with horses, and along pastures owned by the University of Arizona. You're still within city limits, but the density is a bit less.

The connecting bike-and-pedestrian bridge will lead to the landscaped bike paths along the north side of the Rillito River (see separate entry). When the bridge is completed, cyclists will have at least 8 miles of contiguous bike path/bike lane.

Food Facilities Nearby: None.

Restrooms: None.

Special Precautions: Be aware that this is a bike *lane*, not a bike *path*. You will be separated from the vehicular traffic by 3 feet of buffer, but you will still be pedaling beside traffic that may move at 40 or 50 miles per hour (the legal speed limit is 30 miles per hour).

Best Parking Lot: There is no parking set aside for this facility.

Directions: To get to 2nd Street and Mountain Avenue, the path's beginning: Take the Speedway exit from I-10. Go east several blocks to Mountain Avenue. Turn right. Parking is catch-as-catch-can. On weekends, when the university is less busy, parking is easier. During the week, you might have problems.

For More Information: Alternative Modes Coordinator, City of Tucson, Department of Transportation, P.O. Box 27210, Tucson, Arizona 85726-7210. Tel.: (520) 791-4372.

6. Indian Bend Wash and Camelback Walk

General Description:

A 12-mile path snaking through exquisitely land-scaped urban parkland, following the contours of the park's small hills, including lushly exotic trees and shrubs, golf courses, and well-maintained flower gardens.

Level of Difficulty: Easy to average.

Type of Scenery: Golf courses and urban parkland; several large, man-made lakes; tennis courts, ballfields, and playgrounds; lots of grass and trees; colorful gardens with cascading bougainvillaea; pricey housing developments.

Condition of Pavement: Well-maintained concrete.

General Background:

When it rains in Scottsdale, water pours out of the McDowell Mountains in the northeast and the Phoenix Mountains in the northwest to converge, sometimes violently, in the slough known as Indian Bend Wash. One year in the 1970s, two "hundred year" floods occurred within three months of each other, destroying property and taking many lives.

Scottsdale, a city with some very pricey real estate,

declined the usual solution—channeling the slough with concrete and surrounding it with high wire fencing. The fenced-off channel would have sliced the city in half, would have been incredibly ugly, and would have wasted too much valuable land.

Instead, designers created an unusual greenbelt of public parks, golf courses, swimming pools, and small lakes that doubled as a flood-control system. Rather than deepening and concretizing the slough, designers planted deep-rooted grass that resisted erosion. Trees and shrubs were planted where they would not be easily uprooted and washed downstream.

Playgrounds, fishing ponds, and tennis courts dot the corridor, and a bike path runs the greenbelt's 12-mile length. No one in the city is more than a few moments' walk away from the parkland. Proud of the achievement, city officials are extending the recreational system. Scottsdale has recently annexed a considerable amount of land directly north of the city center. Throughout this newly acquired area will run a greenbelt and bike path. By the turn of the century, this path may be 30 miles long.

The Bike Path:

You can pick up the path in Tempe, near the intersection of Hayden Road and the Salt River, but most people think of Indian Bend Wash as beginning at the Scottsdale/Tempe border. This begins on McKellips road, between Miller and Hayden Roads (McClintock Road in Tempe).

You'll begin the ride by seeing McKellips Lake Park, an 18-acre park offering fishing, picnicking, and sailing.

Next you'll come to the 52-acre Vista del Camino Park, with a series of smaller ponds. This community center offers baseball and basketball as well as fishing and picnicking.

Crossing McDowell Road, you'll come to the 8-acre McDowell Exhibit Plaza. Community programs are held here. Some of the concrete structures are flood-control tools designed to direct water flow. North of the plaza is the 55-acre El Dorado Park, with more ponds and sports facilities.

After crossing Oak Street you come to the Thomas Rest Stop, designed for bicyclists. There are restrooms and water, several picnic tables under shady shelters, and several bike racks.

Continuing north, you'll ride through several privately developed golf courses. Underpasses take you beneath both Indian School Road and Camelback Road. You'll ride through Indian School Park, a well-developed city park where you'll find, among other amenities, the Indian Bend Wash Information Center. In this park there are also sports fields and public facilities, including tennis courts especially designed to break away and float during floods. When the waters recede, the courts return to their foundations, undamaged.

Next comes another golf course and then Chaparral Park. This park has a huge lake with great fishing (the city stocks it) and a free-form public swimming pool.

North of Indian School Road the path tends to stay close to busy Hayden Road, but it remains an attractive, comfortable, and interesting ride. Transportation officials are improving some sections of the path by widening the buffer between path and roadway. You'll cross the Arizona Canal (see separate entry), Indian Bend Road, and then McCormick Parkway.

At this point, technically speaking, you are no longer in Indian Bend Wash but along Camelback Walk. You'll be riding past expensive homes with luscious cascades of red-ripe bougainvillaea, past restaurants with outdoor cafes overlooking the bike path and small ponds, and on into areas that are only beginning to be developed.

Out in this northern, somewhat hillier section of the city, the paths will ultimately fork off in many different directions. For example, north of Via Linda, you'll ride through Mountain View Park. Several underpasses later, you can turn right onto Mountain View Road, leaving the bike path to ride on the street for a short distance of just over a mile, until you reach the Scottsdale Ranch Park path with its additional several miles of bike paths.

More such choices will become available as the city grows. Scottsdale is insisting that developers include bike-path extensions and connections throughout their properties.

Food Facilities Nearby: Many good sandwich shops and restaurants all along the length of the path.

Restrooms: The Mustang Library; Mountain View Park; Chaparral Park; Indian School Park; Civic Center area; El Dorado Park; McDowell Park; Vista del Camino Park.

Special Precautions: This path is somewhat narrow. It is a recreational path, meant for leisurely cycling. Don't expect to ride at high speeds.

There are a few difficult road crossings here, but most have been eliminated by underpasses. The city is working on the problem.

Best Parking Lot: Thomas Bike Stop Rest Area.

Directions: To get to the southern beginning of Indian Bend Wash, take Route 60 exit off I-10. Drive several miles and turn left onto McClintock Road in Tempe. After several miles, McClintock will cross the Salt River. Turn left on McKellips Road and look for the bike path.

For the Thomas Bike Stop Rest Area: Continue along McClintock Road (at the Tempe/Scottsdale boundary, the name will change to Hayden Road). After several miles, turn left onto Thomas Road. Look for the rest area.

For More Information: The City of Scottsdale, Transportation Department, P.O. Box 1000, 7447 East Indian School Road, Suite 205, Scottsdale, Arizona 85252. Tel.: (602) 994-2732.

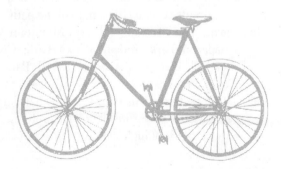

7. The Crosscut Canal and Papago Park

SCOTTSDALE, ARIZONA

General Description:

A 3-mile flat canal-side path leading into Papago Park's extensive network of paved and unpaved cycling paths.

Level of Difficulty: Easy canal-side path; park paths vary in difficulty.

Type of Scenery: Urban backyards; mature salt cedars along the canal path; open, rolling hills in Papago Park with saguaro cacti and mesquite bosques.

Condition of Pavement: Good.

General Background:

Papago Park, one of the nation's largest city parks, has several ponds with picnic areas, the nearby Phoenix Zoo, and the Desert Botanical Garden with exhibits of arid-region plants from around the world.

If you have any interest at all in plants, plan to spend several hours at the botanical garden, enjoying the variety of exhibits. "Plants and People of the Sonoran Desert" is a 3-acre exhibit of ancient and modern desert life. The Desert House Information and Technical Center explores state-of-the-art, energy-conscious home construction. One branch of the Papago Park bike path leads to the botanical garden, where you can tour and have lunch.

The Bike Path:

To begin riding on the Crosscut Canal's paved path, you'll need to cross over the canal from Osborn Road on a pedestrian bridge. The canal-side ride will be through residential areas, under soothing corridors of tall and shady salt cedars. You'll skirt an industrial area and the city's automobile-dealer row. An underpass will help you cross McDowell Road, a major street.

Next you'll come to the northern entrance to Papago Park. The paths branch here so you can choose to head west to the center of the park with its ponds and picnic areas, or east to the botanical garden and zoo. Once you enter the park, many paths branch off from the main route. Following the central path will take you to the Salt River, south of the park.

For the Avid Cyclist: Papago Park is a mountain-biking mecca with short, steep climbs over rocks and hills and a vast network of dirt trails, varying from easy to difficult.

Food Facilities Nearby: Snack areas at the zoo and garden.

Restrooms: In the center of Papago Park; the zoo; the entrance to the botanical garden.

Special Precautions: Drink lots of water, and ride with a friend in this urban area.

Best Parking Lot: Papago Park.

Directions: To Papago Park, from I-10, take Route 60 East.

Almost immediately, turn north (left) onto Priest Drive. After 3 miles, cross the Salt River and enter the park.

The north end of the Crosscut Canal is near the intersection of Osborn and Scottsdale Roads.

For More Information: The City of Scottsdale, Transportation Department, P.O. Box 1000, 7447 East Indian School Road, Suite 205, Scottsdale, Arizona 85252. Tel.: (602) 994-2732.

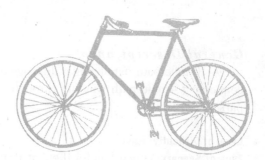

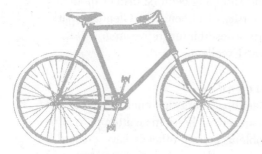

8. The Arizona Canal Diversion Channel and the Thunderbird Paseo

PHOENIX AND GLENDALE, ARIZONA

General Description:

A 10-mile path paralleling a drainage channel, and a connecting 4-mile path winding through a grassy linear park.

Level of Difficulty: Easy.

Type of Scenery: Very urban for the first 10 miles—walled-in backyards and shopping centers; distant mountain views; the University of Phoenix. In Glendale, parks and tennis courts; a desert interpretive area.

Condition of Pavement: Excellent.

General Background:

The cities of Maricopa County are encroaching on the desert at the rate of an acre an hour. In an attempt to mitigate the traffic problem, county officials have created a 400-mile bikeways system that includes on-street striped bike lanes and an extensive network of bike paths. Look for an additional 20 or 30 miles in the next few years.

The county has been able to develop so much mileage so quickly by taking advantage of the two separate water systems: the canals that bring water into the area, and the drainage systems that take the water away. The irrigation canals were here long before the cities. The very sophisticated Hohokam people, expert farmers, built them centuries ago. Some of the drainage system—the creeks and washes and riverbeds—is the work of nature. The rest is the work of modern man.

This includes the Arizona Canal Diversion Channel (the ACDC), a boxed and paved channel that widens gradually as it travels out of the center of Phoenix, passes through the city, and opens into an uncontained grassy wash called the Thunderbird Paseo.

Along this drainage waterway the county has built a bike path, including numerous underpasses, *each* costing from $750,000 to $1 million.

The Bike Path:

The ACDC begins on the west side of 24th Street in Phoenix, just south of the Phoenix Mountain Preserve and north of Camelback Road. It heads northwest, paralleling the mountains for about 6 miles. When the mountains end, the drainage canal heads more directly west until it reaches Glendale and widens out into the natural wash.

The ACDC closely parallels the Arizona Canal, a water *import* system. For a short section the ACDC actually goes underground in order to avoid crossing some school property. At this point the ACDC temporarily diverts to the Arizona Canal, passing under shady stands of mature mesquite trees. After the school property, the ACDC comes back aboveground and the bike path returns to it.

West of the Phoenix Mountains the path passes several universities, including the University of Phoenix, then passes underneath I-17. West of I-17 is a large shopping development with a huge amusement park, Castles and Coasters, recognizable by its lavishly colorful loop-the-loop roller coaster.

Soon after, the canal reaches the city limits of Glendale. West of the border, the path changes names and style. It's now called the Thunderbird Paseo. Glendale chose to develop this 4-mile section into a greenway filled with recreational facilities, similar to Indian Bend Wash (see separate entry). Thunderbird Paseo, wide and grassy, has lots of sports areas and places for people to relax.

Food Facilities Nearby: Sandwich shops and restaurants at many intersections along the path's length.

Restrooms: At each park in Glendale.

Special Precautions: Go slowly through the underpasses. There have been a few serious collisions.

At the several difficult aboveground road crossings, officials would like cyclists to walk their bikes.

Best Parking Lot: In Glendale, a parking area within the Paseo, near the intersection of 59th Avenue and Thunderbird Road. (Along the ACDC, parking is catch-as-catch can.)

Directions: From I-17, take the Thunderbird Road exit. Head west to 59th Avenue. Turn left onto 59th. One short city block later, you'll see the park on your right.

For More Information: The City of Glendale Traffic Engineering Department, 5850 West Glendale Avenue, Glendale, Arizona 85301. Tel.: (602) 435-4163.

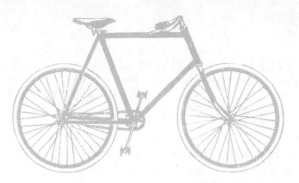

The City of Phoenix Street Transportation Department, 200 West Washington Street, 5th Floor, Phoenix, Arizona 85003-1611. Tel.: (602) 262-1650.

The Bicycle Program of the Transportation Planning Division, Maricopa County Department of Transportation, 2901 W. Durango Street, Phoenix, Arizona 85009. Tel.: (602) 506-3994.

 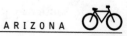

9. Dreamy Draw Park

General Description:

A 3-mile path winding up and down the hills of a desert mountain park.

Level of Difficulty: Challenging.

Type of Scenery: Open desert parkland; saguaro cacti and other distinctive Sonoran Desert vegetation; hilly land with some long, fairly steep grades.

Condition of Pavement: Good.

The Bike Path:

Dreamy Draw Park, one of several minimally developed parks within the extensive Phoenix Mountains Preserve, is only moments away from the urban hubbub. If you're tired of the city, this is the place to ride. You'll coast among forests of 10-foot-high saguaro cactus, far from buildings and crowds, in a place of respite that is accessible by bike from the Arizona Canal Diversion Channel (ACDC)/Thunderbird Paseo (see separate entry).

The bed of this bike path used to be a narrow automobile road. As the city grew northward, traffic through the mountains increased and the city built a four-lane highway through the mountain preserve.

The old two-lane road became a 12-foot-wide north-to-south bike path with a downhill grade into the city center. The dirt paths branching off the paved path are open to experienced mountain cyclists.

At the southern end of Dreamy Draw, the path ends at a $400,000 bike-and-pedestrian bridge that helps you across a busy automobile road. To get to the ACDC (see separate entry), cross the bridge and go south on Dreamy Draw Road. Turn right onto Glendale Avenue. Go west (you can ride on sidewalks in this city) until you reach the eastern end of the ACDC, about a mile away.

For the Avid Cyclist: These two paths combined make a good day's ride. Park at the staging area in the Thunderbird Paseo (see separate entry), ride the Thunderbird Paseo/ACDC to Glendale Avenue. Take the short, on-street jog to the Dreamy Draw bridge and ride up through the park. If you return along the same route, you'll have ridden more than 30 miles, mostly on bike paths, and enjoyed a fair amount of scenic variety.

Food Facilities Nearby: None.

Restrooms: At staging area.

Special Precautions: This path is very hilly, very hot, and generally shadeless. Bring plenty of water. Don't ride in the middle of the day, unless you are used to desert heat.

There is a downhill grade to this path, from north to south.

Ride with a friend in this isolated city park.

Best Parking Lot: The Phoenix Mountains Preserve staging area.

Directions: Dreamy Draw Park is one of several city parks within the Phoenix Mountains Preserve, also called the North Mountain Preserve. The park is accessed off the east end of Northern Avenue. From I-17, take the Northern Avenue exit and head east. Follow it for several miles until it dead-ends in the park.

For More Information: The City of Phoenix Transportation Department, 200 West Washington Street, 5th Floor, Phoenix, Arizona 85003-1611. Tel.: (602) 262-1650.

The Bicycle Program of the Transportation Planning Division, Maricopa County Department of Transportation, 2901 W. Durango Street, Phoenix, Arizona 85009. Tel.: (602) 506-3994.

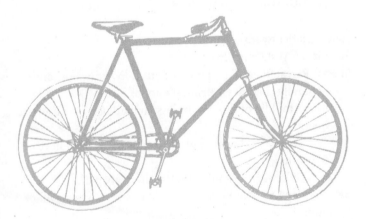

10. The Rio Salado Project

General Description:

Currently, 1 mile along the south bank and 1 mile along the north bank of the Salt River, with several miles to be added yearly.

Level of Difficulty: Very easy.

Type of Scenery: Landscaped and developed lakes; upscale urban development of stores, restaurants, sports arenas; riding stable and large city park nearby.

Condition of Pavement: Excellent.

General Background:

This tiny nugget of bike path promises, within the next several years, to expand into a world-class biking facility. The ultimate plan is for a 20-mile-long recreational and biking greenway following the Salt River, a plan likely to come to fruition after the turn of the century.

The Rio Salado Project will be a center for outdoor activity. When you're done riding you'll be able to take your pick of a number of cafes and restaurants strung out along the waterway. Eventually, there will be a string of lakes with boating opportunities.

Another 3.5 miles along the south bank will be built well before the decade's end, and 14 more miles will be completed soon after.

The Bike Path:

The 2 miles, parallel segments along the north and south banks of the Salt River, are just the beginning. These parallel paths extend from Mill Avenue to Rural Road. On the north side of the river the path connects to the Indian Bend Wash path (see separate entry) and the trail facilities in Papago Park (see separate entry).

You will get from the south bank to the north bank on the Mill Avenue Bridge. There is no special bike path on the bridge, but you may ride on the sidewalk, in the direction of vehicular traffic.

Food Facilities Nearby: To be developed.

Restrooms: To be developed.

Special Precautions: None.

Best Parking Lot: To be developed.

Directions: From I-10, take the exit for Highway 60. Go east. Almost immediately, turn left onto Priest Drive. Go north until you reach the Rio Salado. Parking is currently catch-as-catch-can on city streets.

For More Information: The City of Tempe, Public Works Department, P.O. Box 5002, Tempe, Arizona 85280. Tel.: (602) 350-8204.

The Bicycle Program of the Transportation Planning Division, Maricopa County Department of Transportation, 2901 W. Durango Street, Phoenix, Arizona 85009. Tel.: (602) 506-3994.

11. Rio de Flag Canyon and the Sinclair Wash

General Description:

A 4.5-mile trail beginning in a large county park, passing under extensive stands of ponderosa pine, and winding through an undeveloped canyon near the city center.

Level of Difficulty: Average.

Type of Scenery: High-country evergreen forests; great views of snowcapped mountains; riparian habitat in the canyon; parkland; some urban development; a short stretch near a busy road.

Condition of Pavement: Packed aggregate, suitable for most roadbikes except those with very narrow tires; prey to washouts during spring flooding.

General Background:

The city of Flagstaff (population about 50,000) is the outdoor center of northern Arizona. People come for cross-country and downhill skiing, hiking and camping, mountain biking, river rafting, rock climbing and caving.

This is a young city. Its name comes from the 1876 centennial, when people cut down a ponderosa pine and hung a flag on it. Flagstaff has been on the map for a century, but (until a decade or so ago) you'd have missed it if you'd blinked as you drove through town.

This is also a high-country city. At nearly 7,000 feet, it's one of the highest urban areas in the continental United States, and the surrounding peaks stand 3,000, 4,000, or 5,000 feet above the city itself. At these altitudes, the desert has yielded to green forests and open grasslands.

In 1990, the city began to build a five-pronged network of urban bike paths allowing cyclists to ride through the city and out to most of the surrounding forestlands.

The Rio de Flag Canyon trail, near the city center, is the system's keystone trail. All the other bike paths will eventually connect to this one. This visionary system is both an effective transportation system *and* a beautiful ride. The system is one of the most naturally beautiful in the country.

The Bike Path:

The trail begins in the county park, Fort Tuthill, in Flagstaff's southwest corner. The first 3 miles follow a narrow-gauge logging railroad bed. There are soft and gentle grades and cool pine forests, perfect for young children or for older adults who want to avoid difficult hills.

Leaving the park, you'll pass a few scattered houses and the small village of Mountain Dell, then cross Sinclair Wash on several pretty little bike bridges. Next, the trail briefly parallels a busy highway, although not too closely, then winds through the 15,000-student campus of Northern Arizona University. The campus segment is more difficult.

When you cross Lone Tree Road (a busy road, despite

its name) via an underpass, the trail's name changes from the Sinclair Wash to the Rio de Flag. This 1.5-mile segment passes through a narrow canyon. Above, the hustle-and-bustle urban beat goes on, but all you'll hear down in the canyon is the wind in the pines and the distant whistle of a train. Narrow dirt footpaths branch off the main trail and switchback up the canyon walls.

The canyon trail currently ends at Babbitt Way. By decade's end it will connect with the McMillan Mesa trail (see separate entry) and the Rio de Flag North Trail (see separate entry).

Food Facilities Nearby: None.

Restrooms: Fort Tuthill County Park.

Special Precautions: If you ride here in early spring, check with city hall on the path's condition. Some sections are prone to washouts from spring meltwater.

Best Parking Lot: Fort Tuthill County Park.

Directions: Fort Tuthill Park is adjacent to I-17. From I-17, take Exit 337, the interchange for the airport. Go west, driving directly into the park.

A loop road goes through the park. The trail entrance is on the northwest corner of the loop, near the horse racetrack.

All Flagstaff's bike paths in this system are well marked with the system logo: a small, discreet sign that says "Urban Trail System." The entrances to each trail are also marked by attractive post-and-split-rail fencing.

For More Information: The City of Flagstaff Planning Division, 211 West Aspen Avenue, Flagstaff, Arizona 86001. Tel.: (520) 779-7632.

12. The Observatory Mesa Trail

General Description:

A 2-mile path through forest-filled parkland using switchbacks to climb a steep mesa, with terrific views on top in all directions, including a distant view of the North Rim of the Grand Canyon.

Level of Difficulty: Very challenging.

Type of Scenery: City parkland; evergreen forests; terrific long-distance views from the top of the mesa; access to the unpaved trail system of the Forest Service.

Condition of Pavement: Packed, crushed aggregate, usually suitable for roadbikes but subject to washouts.

General Background:

This segment of Flagstaff's Urban Trail System is anything but "urban." From the trail's beginning in Thorpe Park, the forestland beckons; you'll quickly leave the buildings and the noise of city life far below.

The privately run Lowell Observatory owns this property. Percival Lowell, born in 1855 of the illustrious Lowells of Boston, was the first astronomer to theorize the existence of a planet beyond Neptune. Pluto was discovered in 1930, almost 15 years after Lowell's death. Lowell is equally famous for a second theory: that Mars was inhabited, as evidenced by the lines Lowell saw in his telescope and which he said were canals. Lowell's observatory has been operational since 1894.

Observatory and city officials have worked out access agreements allowing cyclists to cross observatory property to get to Forest Service trails on the other side of the mesa. Cyclists are asked to stay on the trails and not explore the limits of the observatory's property.

The Bike Path:

The path begins below the mesa in Thorpe Park. The climb up onto the mesa through thick pine forests begins gently but soon becomes quite steep. There are several switchbacks—unusual for an urban bike path. Don't give up. The view is worth the effort.

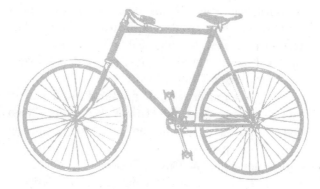

 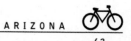

Atop the mesa, your second mile will be easier. The thick forests thin out. If you're lucky, you can see the North Rim of the Grand Canyon. You wouldn't call the mile across the mesa "flat," but after the haul up those switchbacks, it might seem easy.

In Thorpe Park, where the path begins, there is an intersection with the Rio de Flag North (see separate entry).

For the Avid Cyclist: Across the mesa, you'll find the national forest's dirt trails, for experienced mountain cyclists.

Food Facilities Nearby: None.

Restrooms: Thorpe Park.

Special Precautions: This is a very steep climb. Be prepared.

Best Parking Lot: Thorpe Park.

Directions: From I-40, take Exit 195. Go north. In Flagstaff this becomes Milton Road. The road passes under railroad tracks and bends sharply to the right. Don't go to the right. Turn left onto Santa Fe Avenue. Drive west 5 blocks to Thorpe Road. Turn right and drive a short distance on Thorpe Road.

The bike trail crosses Thorpe Road and is marked by both the sign with the "Urban Trail System" logo and the post-and-split-rail fencing. Across from the trail is a large parking lot.

For More Information: The City of Flagstaff Planning Division, 211 West Aspen Avenue, Flagstaff, Arizona 86001. Tel.: (520) 779-7632.

13. Rio de Flag North

General Description:

A 2.5-mile path that will extend another 1.5 miles by the end of 1996. The path begins in the city's northwest corner at Schultz Pass and vaguely parallels the Fort Valley Road, terminating at the city center or branching off onto the Observatory Mesa Trail.

Level of Difficulty: Easy to average.

Type of Scenery: The banks of the Rio de Flag; suburban backyards; pretty city parkland and school property; a mile north of city hall, a large open area and a pond.

Condition of Pavement: Packed crushed aggregate.

The Bike Path:

By the end of 1996, this trail will be about 4 miles long, extending from Schultz Pass, in the city's northwest corner, down into the city center. This generally downhill ride follows the course of the Rio de Flag as it tumbles out of the San Francisco Peaks. From Schultz Pass (where you can access Forest Service dirt trails), as you ride toward the city you'll cross Highway 180, the road to the Grand Canyon.

Continuing south, you'll ride through property managed by the Museum of Northern Arizona, a top-flight regional museum featuring exhibits on local geology, paleontology, and cultural history. You'll cross the Rio de Flag on a bike bridge and wind down the hillside through forested areas. You'll ride briefly through a suburban area with backyards and high fencing.

Passing through Thorpe Park, you'll come to a small pond. Near this pond is the intersection with the Observatory Mesa Trail (see separate entry). By following the Rio de Flag from Schultz Pass and then turning onto Observatory Mesa, you'll ride about 6 miles of contiguous bike path, mostly through stands of pine and open meadowland.

If you don't turn off onto Observatory Mesa, you'll continue on the Rio de Flag North to its in-town terminus, Wheeler Park, a small square in the city center near city hall.

Food Facilities Nearby: None.

Restrooms: Thorpe Park.

Special Precautions: None.

Best Parking Lot: Wheeler Park; Thorpe Park; at the north end of the trail—no official parking area, catch-as-catch-can.

Directions: To Thorpe Park: From I-40, take Exit 195. Go north, into Flagstaff. This becomes Milton Road. After a mile, the road passes under a railroad bridge and bends sharply to the right. Don't go to the right. Turn left onto Santa Fe Avenue. Drive west 5 blocks to Thorpe Road. Turn right. Drive a short distance on Thorpe Road.

The trail crosses Thorpe Road. It will be marked by both the sign with the "Urban Trail System" logo and the post-and-split-rail fencing. Across from the trail is a large parking lot.

To Wheeler Park: When you pass under the railroad tracks, the road ends to the right and becomes Route 66. Take this road. Drive 1 block to Humphries, also called U.S. 180, the road to the Grand Canyon. Turn onto Humphries and go 1 block. Turn left onto Aspen. There will be a large city parking lot. The bike path begins there.

For More Information: The City of Flagstaff Planning Division, 211 West Aspen Avenue, Flagstaff, Arizona 86001. Tel.: (520) 779-7632.

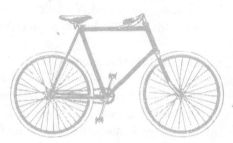

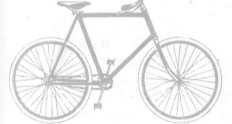

 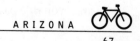

14. Buffalo Park and McMillan Mesa

General Description:

A 3-mile path traversing a mesa escarpment, then connecting with a 3-mile loop that circles a large park where buffalo once grazed. A 1-mile side spur descends from the mesa to a housing development below.

Level of Difficulty: Average.

Type of Scenery: Views of the dramatic San Francisco Peaks; forested areas; parkland; views out over the city; you can see almost 360 degrees from various points on the path to distant mesas and buttes.

Condition of Pavement: Packed crushed aggregate.

The Bike Path:

This trail will eventually connect with the Rio de Flag Canyon trail (see separate entry) near Babbitt Way, in the hub of the city. You'll be able to ride all the way from Fort Tuthill Park in the southwest corner of the city to Buffalo Park, in the northeast corner. Look for this completing link to be built near the end of the decade.

If you want a fairly easy ride that's outside of the city, this is the path for you. From the Buffalo Park staging area, you ride past the huge statue of a buffalo, through the park gates, and into the park itself. You can go either to the right or to the left. It really doesn't matter; you'll be riding a loop around the park, along the rim of the mesa. This path is mostly out in the open, under scattered stands of trees and through alpine meadowland. It's mostly flat, but you'll encounter one short drop and a steep climb as you ride into a draw and up the other side.

When you finish the loop, you'll have returned to the parking area. At the other side of this parking lot, a 3-mile-long path runs along McMillan Mesa, a piece of property adjacent to Buffalo Park and owned by the city. Since the path runs along the edge of an escarpment, you'll get some terrific views of Flagstaff below and of forests 50 miles to the east. Unless you like rugged mountain biking, you'll have to double back along the same path to return to the parking lot.

Food Facilities Nearby: None.
Restrooms: Port-o-potties at Buffalo Park.
Special Precautions: None.
Best Parking Lot: Buffalo Park.
Directions: From I-40, take Exit 195. Go north into Flagstaff. This becomes Milton Road. After more than a mile, the road passes under a railroad bridge and bends sharply to the right, becoming Route 66. Follow Route 66 for 2 blocks. Turn left onto Beaver Street. Go north a little more than a mile. At the stoplight, turn right onto Forest. Stay on that road for more than a mile, as the road climbs up to the top of the mesa. Go left onto Gemini Drive. This road leads straight into the park.
For More Information: The City of Flagstaff Planning Division, 211 West Aspen Avenue, Flagstaff, Arizona 86001. Tel.: (520) 779-7632.

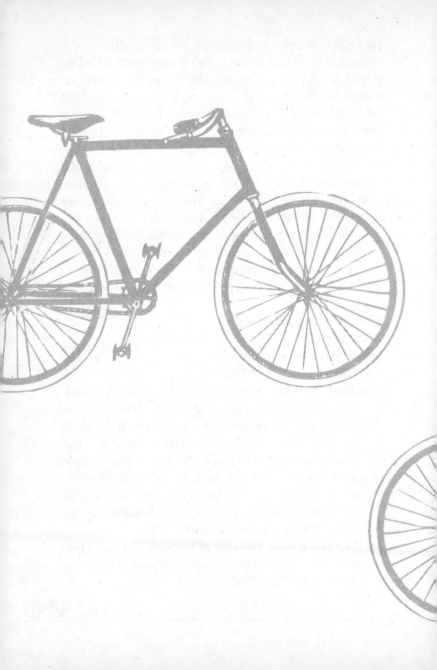

Northern
California

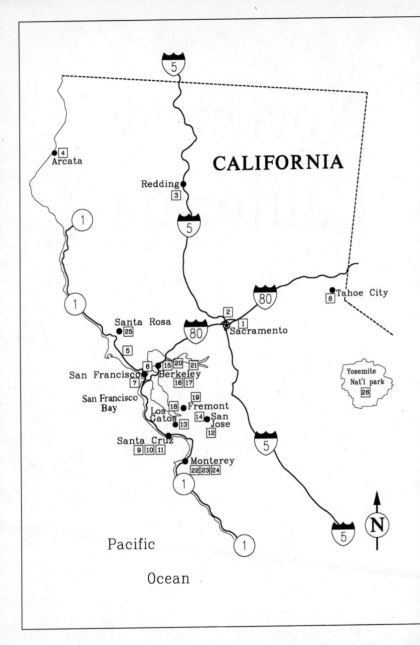

Northern California

1. The American River Parkway

SACRAMENTO TO FOLSOM, CALIFORNIA

General Description:

The granddaddy of all bikeways! A 32.8-mile path running through wetlands, conservation lands, and well-preserved riparian riverbank, extending from the confluence of the American and Sacramento Rivers up to Folsom Dam.

Level of Difficulty: Average.

Type of Scenery: Historic Old Sacramento, with its railroad museum and statue commemorating the western endpoint of the Pony Express; public parklands that include swimming, boating, picnic, and recreation areas; sandbars for wading, shallow ponds for fishing, campgrounds for overnight stays; few road crossings and few residential areas; birdlife and wildlife and warnings to watch out for mountain lions.

Condition of Pavement: Excellent.

General Background:

During California's gold frenzy, so many men panned for gold along the American River that, in only a few years, the river's shape, depth, and flow were forever altered. Today telltale mounds of pebbles from the riverbed are everywhere, looking like ominous burial mounds. Long piles of tailings parallel the riverbank like miniature mountain ranges.

Gold mining altered the region's history as well as its topography. Sacramento, which might otherwise have remained a ranching town, became the new state's capital because it was a hub for the gold-mining industry. The gold-based economic boom lured an educated populace with a predilection for new ideas and technology—as in the bicycle.

Thus began the Sacramento Wheelmen, the state's first bicycle club. The Wheelmen built the Capital City Wheelway, a Sacramento-to-Folsom cinder path. When the wheelway opened on April 12, 1896, about 500 cyclists joined in the celebration. Today's bikeway evolved from that century-old path. Officially named the "Jedediah Smith Memorial Bicycle Trail," after an explorer who camped along the river in 1827, the path today is usually just called the American River Parkway.

This is a bikes-only paved path, one of the few nationwide. Skaters are not permitted. Equestrians have a separate dirt trail. We've heard that Sacramento County is cutting back its park budget, but officials told us not to worry. The bikeway tops the priority list. We're not surprised, since this riverway is an obvious economic asset. Many hotels along the bikeway, for example, lure clientele by providing free bikes.

Currently under construction is a project which will create a 61-mile paved-path loop that will include the American River bikeway, the Sacramento Northern (see separate entry), and the Dry Creek Parkway, currently in the planning stage. The county is also building several smaller feeder paths that will branch off the American River path.

The Bike Path:

The American River bikeway western terminus is in Old Sacramento, near the endpoint of the Pony Express. If you have the time, walk around for an hour. You'll see the Delta King (an old riverboat that's now a hotel), an old railroad station, the California State Railroad Museum, and much more.

For a short distance riding along the path, you'll be biking along the Sacramento River, but quite soon you'll cross the American River on a bridge and head east along that river's north bank.

Next the path winds through Discovery Park, a city park within the river's floodplain. Here, during the spring, the path may be covered with water. Within Discovery Park, the path remains close to the river for about a mile and then drifts over to the park's outermost edge.

Although you won't see the river for much of the length of the bikeway, you'll be enjoying its blessings. Only 4 percent of California's original riparian habitat remains; the rest has been buried under housing developments and office parks. The 5,000 riparian acres in the American River Parkway represent a substantial proportion of what's left.

Within the riverway, an exceptional variety of species thrive. Extremely water-dependent trees like willow and Fremont cottonwood grow along the riverbanks, where their roots are routinely bathed in flowing water. More distant from the wet banks are more drought-resistant trees like interior live oaks and blue oaks. Mixed in among those are digger pines, evergreens found more frequently in the foothill elevations. Many imported species mix with the California natives, although park botanists hope gradually to eliminate these exotic influences.

Continuing east along the trail, you'll see signs warning of mountain lion. In the 1920s, biologists believed about 600 mountain lions remained in California. By the 1970s, estimates had risen to 2,000, and then again to about 6,000 by the mid-1990s. The social status of mountain lions has also been raised. Called "bountied predators" until 1963, hunters were paid for each lion killed. In 1969, the lion's status rose to "game mammal," and in 1990 to "special protected mammal."

The farther east you ride, the more rugged the terrain becomes. The snowcapped Sierras loom larger, the water in the river flows faster, and the hills become steeper. A few climbs in this section have grades of 5 percent or even 7 percent. Although the ride east from Sacramento is generally uphill, you probably won't feel your quadriceps burn until you near Folsom.

The easternmost 8 miles of path, through state-park lands, may feel somewhat isolated at times. You'll pass under shady canopies of trees draped with a jungle-like thickness of tangled vines and shrubs and underbrush. At other times you'll ride through open meadows with wildflowers and soaring hawks. You'll see Folsom Prison with its ominous turret and barbed wire on your right, and then Folsom Dam.

Finally you'll cross the Sacramento/Placer county line,

entering the heart of gold-rush country. The bike trail ends at Beals Point on Folsom Lake. If you're making the return trip, this is a good rest stop. Folsom Lake has picnic, boating, and swimming areas, restrooms, water, a large parking lot, and overnight camping.

Food Facilities Nearby: Old Sacramento; nothing else near the trail, so bring plenty of food and drink.

Restrooms: Along the first third of this ride, restrooms are surprisingly few. Discovery Park is the westernmost public restroom. After you cross Howe Avenue, about a third of the length of the path, you'll find them every 3 or 4 miles.

Special Precautions: Do not ride this path alone. There have been several rapes along this corridor.

Discovery Park is known for its high rate of automobile thefts. Don't leave valuables in your car. Don't leave bikes unattended, even if they're locked.

The speed limit along the bike trail is 15 miles per hour.

Bicycles are not permitted on the parkway's unpaved trail.

Best Parking Lot: There are many parking areas along this route. Discovery Park, the most popular, has safety and theft problems. Avoid it if you can.

If possible, leave your car at your hotel and bike to the path. You might also consider parking in Old Sacramento.

Folsom Lake State Park is a relatively safe place to park.

Directions: To Discovery Park: From Interstate 5, take the

Garden Highway exit. Go east. Look immediately for signs to Discovery Park.

To Folsom Lake: From Highway 50, take the Folsom Boulevard exit. Go east. Cross the river. Turn right (east) onto Folsom/Auburn Road. You'll see signs for Folsom Dam, and then for Folsom Lake.

For More Information: Sacramento County Parks, 3711 Branch Center Road, Sacramento, California 95827. Tel.: (916) 366-2061.

Folsom Lake State Recreation Area, 7806 Folsom/Auburn Road, Folsom, California 95630. Tel.: (916) 988-0205.

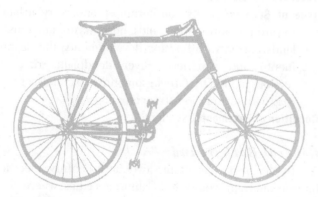

 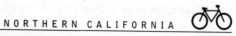

2. The Sacramento Northern Railroad Trail

SACRAMENTO AND RIO LINDA, CALIFORNIA

General Description:

A 5-mile rail trail projected to extend 10.4 miles before the decade's end, with connections to the American River Parkway.

Level of Difficulty: Very easy.

Type of Scenery: At its southernmost end, very urban; toward the north, open fields, horse farms, and grasslands, mixed with housing developments; the Sacramento and American River floodplain; riparian sections along Dry Creek; sometimes parallels a busy road with several side-street crossings.

Condition of Pavement: Excellent.

General Background:

In the beginning of the twentieth century, electric inter-urban trains connected California's cities, where distances were great and road systems undeveloped. The inter-urbans, products of creative engineering, combined city-style trolley cars with long-distance railroad technology. Like trolleys, inter-urbans were powered by overhead electric lines and ran on unobtrusive tracks that allowed passage over major city thoroughfares. But like steam-powered trains, inter-urbans were pulled by large locomotives that could reach speeds of 70 miles an hour outside city limits.

The Sacramento Northern Railroad, among the best of the inter-urbans, ran east from San Francisco to Sacramento, then north to Chico, in the Upper Sacramento Valley. The train allowed the people of Chico to enjoy a day's excursion to sophisticated San Francisco and be home by midnight.

The railroad's final run was on March 1, 1957. Ben Pugh, a bikeways engineer, dug up this *Oakland Tribune* obituary: "The Old Sacramento Northern Railway made its last run of its 44-year career from Oakland as the slanting rain beat a soft requiem on the venerable cars." The tracks lay fallow until rail-trail enthusiasts began building the new path.

The Sacramento Northern connects to the American River bike path (see separate entry) near 12th Street in Sacramento. These two existing bike paths are segments of a proposed 61-mile bikeway loop through the region that is expected to be completed sometime during the first decade of the twenty-first century. Two other proposed segments of the loop are currently in the planning stages.

The Bike Path:

This path begins at its connection to the American River Parkway near 12th Street. The first 0.5 mile runs through the floodplain of the American and Sacramento Rivers along a flood-control levee. Next you'll ride through densely populated areas, crossing several creeks over bike bridges.

Continuing north, the country opens up. By the last mile of the ride, you'll see plenty of horse farms, farmland, meadows, and fields. There's a lengthy stretch that runs beside Dry Creek with its oasis of trees and shrubs. If you're lucky, you'll see beaver, recently returned to these waters because of improved habitat. This used to be an important salmon run. Trail enthusiasts and biologists are working to improve the creek, so more salmon will survive.

Currently the trail ends in Rio Linda. By decade's end there will probably be another 5 miles, extending north to the town of Elverta, passing through a mixture of farmland and developments.

Food Facilities Nearby: None.

Restrooms: None.

Special Precautions: This trail system passes through a major metropolitan center. Ride with a friend.

Best Parking Lot: Rio Linda/Elverta Community Center.

Directions: From Interstate 5, take the Highway 99 exit north to Marysville and Yuba City.

Take the Elkhorn Boulevard exit. Go east, about 7 miles. At the first stoplight, Rio Linda Boulevard, turn left. At the next stop sign, at the Rio Linda Arch, turn right onto "M" Street. Go about 1 mile. Turn right onto Front Street. Follow this street to the community center.

For More Information: The Rio Linda/Elverta Community Center, 810 Oak Lane, Rio Linda, California 95673. Tel.: (916) 991-5929.

3. The Sacramento River Trail System

General Description:

An outstanding ride! This 8-mile, 12-foot-wide river trail uses old gold-mining roads and an 1883 railroad bed to penetrate lush canyon wilderness and includes a sophisticated and graceful stress ribbon bridge, 420 feet long and 13 feet wide—but only 18 inches thick—the first built in North America.

Level of Difficulty: Average.

Type of Scenery: The wilderness along the banks of the Sacramento River; the twists and turns of canyon topography; Redding Arboretum; several city parks and a small science museum; some residential areas.

Condition of Pavement: Excellent.

General Background:

More than 180,000 cubic feet of water per second roared down this canyon riverway during floodtime until the Shasta and Keswick Dams altered the river's wild ways. The gorge carved out by that eons-old raging flow is wide and deep and natural and open. It's a beautiful place to be and a perfect setting for a bikeway.

The city of Redding is sparing no expense, looking

worldwide for the best engineering solutions, in an effort to complement the river's natural beauty. Bikeway planners clearly enjoy considerable support from the people of Redding, who have already contributed more than $1 million in funds and services to the river-trail project.

Soon to be completed is a 60-acre riverside museum, Turtle Bay, and a $3-million bike-and-pedestrian bridge. With both indoor and outdoor exhibits, the museum will emphasize river ecology. The bridge, leading from the 200-acre Redding Arboretum on the river's north bank to the new museum, will be wide enough to allow cyclists to stop and watch the salmon spawn in the river below. Each season—spring, summer, fall, winter—chinook salmon swim as far as the Redding Riffle, the last below the Keswick Dam, to lay their eggs in the gravel and die.

Ultimately the 30-mile system will include paths through commercial centers and the city's extensive park system. Another path, leading to the hotels of Hilltop Drive, will allow tourists to ride down to the river. On the south bank, extensions to Keswick Dam and to Shasta Dam, 13 miles distant, will be built. Paths will also lead to Old Shasta, a state historic park, and into several residential areas.

The Bike Path:

This vastly underrated path is one of the best in California. You might begin from Caldwell Park, on the river's north bank, just east of Diestlehorst Bridge, an automobile bridge with one lane designated as a bikeway. You'll ride east through the arboretum, to enjoy the short-but-sweet natural history trail, with its information plaques placed along the route. Then double back to Caldwell Park (when the Turtle Bay Bridge is ready, you'll cross over and make a loop instead) and ride through a small residential area, which the city hopes to buy.

Then you'll enter our idea of bike-path heaven, a 1.5-mile stretch through some of the most beautiful riverway we've seen. The roller-coaster path tumbles along, rolling easily over the land, complementing the natural surroundings. There *are* some steep hills, but they're short and fun. Most beginning cyclists will have no trouble on a good bike.

Path designers used the old riverbank mining road, so you'll pass several gold mines which made the fortunes or sealed the fates of many hopeful forty-niners. The mine entrances are sealed now, but it's easy to imagine the lives of those men who passed through here 150 years ago.

If you look up, you'll see the stress ribbon bridge—13 feet wide, 420 feet long, but only 18 inches thick. Bikeway designers wanted a bridge with a natural elegance, an artful bridge that complemented the river canyon by being as invisible as possible. The beauty of the Redding bridge lies in its blending with the water and the canyon. A quarter of a mile downstream, the bridge is invisible.

On the south bank of the river, the path uses a Southern Pacific Railroad bed built in 1883. You can turn right and ride toward the Keswick and Shasta Dams, or you can turn left to ride back toward Redding. The path to the dams is a rough, unpaved ride over old railroad ballast. This 13-mile section will be improved within the next few years, as soon as officials find the money for paving, about $100,000 a mile. You can ride quite a distance toward the dams now, but you'll need a fat-tired bike and an enthusiasm for deep gravel.

The path to the left, back to the city, is paved and flatter than the north-bank path. Expect more people. Currently, you can ride about 3 miles along to the Diestlehorst Bridge, an automobile bridge with a designated bike lane that will take you back to Caldwell Park.

Food Facilities Nearby: None.

Restrooms: Caldwell Park.

Special Precautions: Ride with a friend in this semi-wilderness setting.

Best Parking Lot: Caldwell Park.

Directions: From Interstate 5, take the Highway 299/Lake Boulevard exit. Go west. Turn left onto North Market Street/Highway 273. Go down the steep hill toward the river. Turn left onto Quartz Hill Road. You'll enter Caldwell Park. The first parking lot you see will provide the best river-trail access.

For More Information: The City of Redding Parks & Recreation Department, 760 Parkview Avenue, Redding, California 96001-3396. Tel.: (916) 225-4095, or 225-4020.

4. The Hammond Trail

General Description:

A 3-mile, fairly flat recreation path running along the Northern California coast through rustic farmland and open seaside.

Level of Difficulty: Easy.

Type of Scenery: "The Bottoms" farming country with bulb farms, cattle barns, farmhouses, and dairy cows; a converted railroad bridge over the Mad River; ocean, beach, and expanses of dunes and shallow waters; Hiller Park, a community park.

Condition of Pavement: Good.

The Bike Path:

This charming little trail runs through the rich pasturelands at the mouth of the Mad River and along some gentle seashore. We rank it among our top family rides because of its unique combination of great natural beauty and visual variety.

The trail starts at the northern boundary of "The Bottoms," an expanse of flat, rich farmland reminiscent of coastal New England farmland. You'll start at the south end of a logging railroad trestle that crosses the Mad River. The trestle arcs up high above the flowing water and descends next to a cow pasture. Before you start on the bridge, take some time to look at the river below. You're bound to see interesting birdlife—herons, egrets, cormorants, and more—and you may see other animals. Otters and harbor seals enjoy this section of the Mad River.

When you get off the bridge, you may be confused: the bike path and the road are the same. Just keep going straight for a quarter-mile up the hill in front of you. This farming road has some traffic, mostly farm trucks and tractors. As you crest the top of the hill you may encounter residential traffic. You'll pass a general store and ride several blocks.

Past the small store, the bike path begins again. This section is easy riding through some parkland and behind some homes. You'll come to Hiller Park, a community park with picnic tables and restrooms.

Ultimately the path arrives at some exquisite coastal hills. The ocean shoals extend far out to sea, unusual for the Pacific shore. The waves pound the shallows relentlessly, creating white bars of foam as far as the eye can see.

When the bike-path pavement ends, the right-of-way continues for a short distance. Currently it's covered by deep gravel, but is scheduled to be paved quite soon. If you're looking for a quiet place to watch the water, this is the destination for you.

The Hammond Trail continues along the shoreline to a public beach, but there is no bike access. From here on, the trail is limited to horses and walkers.

For the Avid Cyclist: If the Hammond Trail is too short a ride, consider exploring the farming roads that lace the Arcata Bottoms, to the south of the railroad trestle. "The Bottoms," an expanse of several hundred acres of rich farmland, is covered with paved vehicle roads that are sparsely used. You will encounter traffic, but probably not traveling at high speeds. In a poll conducted by the local paper, the *Times-Standard*, the locals voted "The Bottoms" the best place in the area to ride a bike. You can spend a half-day exploring these flat farm roads, riding past the old farmhouses. Some of these fields are filled with flowers as this region grows bulbs for international export.

You can also get to a local public beach from the southern terminus of the Hammond Trail. From the southern end of the railroad trestle, turn west and follow the signs to Mad River Beach.

Food Facilities Nearby: None.

Restrooms: Hiller Park; Mad River Beach.

Special Precautions: This path includes an on-street section. Expect some traffic, but not heavy or fast-moving.

Best Parking Lot: Parking is catch-as-catch-can for this path. You're allowed to park along roadsides in "The Bottoms."

Directions: To the converted railroad trestle, take the Guintoli Lane exit from Highway 101. Go west. Turn right on Janes Road. Turn left onto Iverson Road. Turn right onto Mad River Road. The bridge is on this road.

For More Information: The Humboldt County Parks Department, 1106 Second Street, Eureka, California 95501. Tel.: (707) 445-7650.

5. Samuel P. Taylor State Park and the Golden Gate National Recreation Area

MARIN COUNTY, CALIFORNIA

General Description:

A 5-mile flat trail that runs along a stream that cuts through a canyon, past stands of coastal redwoods and Douglas firs and into the open meadowlands of the Golden Gate National Recreation Area.

Level of Difficulty: Easy.

Type of Scenery: Forestland; a streambed for kids to wade in; in the fall, the spawning of hooked-nose salmon in Papermill Creek.

Condition of Pavement: Good.

General Background:

Samuel Penfield Taylor, a Boston adventurer who won $6,000 in the 1862 gold-rush lottery, bought this hundred acres of timberland along Papermill Creek and began a tourism business that included a resort hotel and a public campground, one of the nation's first.

Now a state park of nearly 3,000 acres, the property continues to provide camping, hiking, and cycling opportunities. The park's ecosystems include wet coastal hillsides, dry canyons and gulches, and lush riverbanks. In the fall, visitors watch the silver salmon spawning runs. Steelhead trout spawn here later in the season.

Since Taylor never logged the land, small groves of old-growth coastal redwoods survive. There are also extensive stands of younger redwoods. Along some of the north-facing slopes you'll see the best of these old redwoods, some with trunks 6 feet in diameter, mixed in with a scattering of deciduous trees.

The Bike Path:

The ride begins in the state park, following the bed of a narrow-gauge railroad along Papermill Creek. About halfway along the length of the trail, when you enter the national recreation area, the forest opens up and you'll bike through flower-filled meadows with intermittent stands of trees. During the summer months people enjoy the bike path because of the adjacent stream, with plenty of places where kids can wade. The park is far enough inland from the ocean to avoid the fog that sometimes diminishes a good bike ride.

This state park has about 60 campsites. Reservations are required from April 1 to October 31; call Mistix at (800) 444-7275.

For the Avid Cyclist: When the paved path ends, there are several more miles of rail trail open to cyclists. However, the additional mileage is unpaved and quite rough.

Food Facilities Nearby: None.

Restrooms: At park headquarters.

Special Precautions: None.

Best Parking Lot: At the state park.

Directions: From Highway 1, in Olema, turn east onto Sir Francis Drake Boulevard. Go about 6 miles. Look for park entrance signs.

For More Information: The Samuel P. Taylor State Park, P.O. Box 251, Lagunitas, California 94938. Tel.: (415) 488-9897.

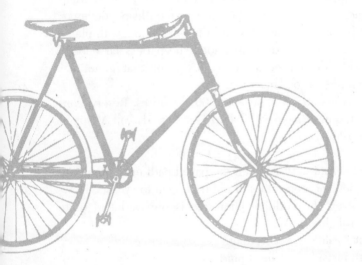

6. Angel Island State Park

General Description:

About 8 miles of paved and unpaved roads, closed to motor vehicles, circle this hilly island, once called "the Ellis Island of the West Coast," in San Francisco Bay.

Level of Difficulty: Average.

Type of Scenery: Decommissioned military base and immigration station; terrific views of San Francisco Bay, including the Golden Gate Bridge and National Recreation Area; a great place to watch the sailboat races in the bay; views of Alcatraz, Treasure Island, and the San Francisco skyline; firings of historic cannon on weekends; Mt. Livermore, more than 750 feet high, from which you can see 40 miles across the bay.

Condition of Pavement: Much of the lower road is paved, but some is packed gravel; the upper fire road is hard-packed dirt, not suitable for most narrow-tired bikes.

General Background:

Angel Island, a hilly and tree-covered parkland, has a rich military history. Beginning about 2,000 years ago, Coastal Miwok Indians visited frequently, paddling from the mainland in their reed boats. When the Spanish arrived, the Miwok left.

The island's superb harbor and location in the bay drew military ships from four different nations over several centuries. After the Spanish came the Russians in 1808, hunting sea otter. In 1814 the British 16-gun sloop the HMS *Raccoon* landed and made emergency repairs. (This is why the deep-water channel between the island and Tiburon is called Raccoon Straight.)

When Mexico ceded California, the United States military arrived. Angel Island was a base of operations for the war waged against the Apache and Sioux. In 1899 a quarantine station treated soldiers who had become ill while serving in the Spanish-American War and in the Philippines. In the twentieth century, the island housed soldiers on their way to serve in the Pacific.

There was also an immigration station, built in 1905 to oversee Asians entering the United States. The station was closed in 1940 and three years later Congress repealed the 60-year-old Chinese Exclusion Act.

In 1963 the island was given to the state of California. With the exception of the Point Blunt and Point Stuart coast guard stations, the entire island is now a state park. There are guided tours through the historic sites and miles of hiking trails as well as biking roads. The water is too rough for swimming. Overnight camping and overnight docking are available by reservation. In-line skating is not permitted. Bicycles may be rented on the island.

The Bike Path:

Two roads at separate elevations circle Angel Island—the fairly flat 5-mile Perimeter Road near sea level and the hilly 3-mile Fire Road at about 450 feet above sea level.

Most families ride the Perimeter Road. When you arrive by boat in Ayala Cove, two paths lead up to the Perimeter Road. The dirt path is for foot traffic only. Park officials do not want bikes on this steep dirt path, because they've added to the erosion problem. A paved path with switchbacks up the 150-foot climb has been built for bikes.

The Perimeter Road passes by several picnic sites and camping areas. When the road traverses the long southern shoreline, it becomes packed gravel, navigable by most road bikes except for those with very narrow tires. The road also passes near most of the historic sites. Bring a bike lock so you can tour these buildings. While this road has no public traffic, you will encounter service vehicles and visitor trams.

The second bike road, the Fire Road, is not suitable for all cyclists. The paved path connecting the lower road and the higher road is quite steep. Be particularly careful when coming *down* the connecting path, since there have been several accidents caused by speeding bikers.

A narrow-tired bike will pose some difficulty on the Fire Road, with its surface of packed dirt. Sometimes the road is smooth, but often it's somewhat rutted and rough. Hybrid and fat-tired bikes ought to be fine. (Bikes are not permitted on any other dirt roads or trails in the park.)

A dirt walking path leads from the Fire Road up to Mt. Livermore, named after the conservationist who led the effort to turn the island into a state park. The peak provides some terrific views of the bay and the city.

Food Facilities Nearby: Sandwiches at the island snack bar.
Restrooms: At the visitor center in Ayala Cove, and at many

other spots along the Perimeter Road; none along the Fire Road.

Special Precautions: Be careful of the few steep grades on the island's biking roads. Pedestrians use these, too.

Poison oak covers the island.

Best Parking Lot: This island is accessible by private boat or by public ferry. Most people catch the ferry from Tiburon.

Directions: To the Tiburon Ferry, from Highway 101 take the Tiburon Boulevard exit. Go east. In Tiburon, look for a small sign near the water that says "Angel Island Parking." The ferry is on Main Street, about a quarter-mile from the parking area.

For More Information: Angel Island State Park, P.O. Box 318, Tiburon, California 94920. Tel.: (415) 435-1915. (For Angel Island brochures, send $2 plus postage.)

For information on ferry service from Tiburon, call the Angel Island State Park Ferry Company in Tiburon. Tel.: (415) 435-2131.

For information on ferry service from San Francisco or Vallejo, call the Red and White Fleet. Tel.: (415) 546-2896 or (800) BAY-CRUISE.

7. Ft. Point Historic Park and the Golden Gate National Recreation Area

SAN FRANCISCO, CALIFORNIA

General Description:

A 3.5-mile, mostly flat path that begins beneath the San Francisco end of the Golden Gate Bridge and follows the man-made shoreline to Aquatic Park.

Level of Difficulty: Very easy (except for one steep hill).
Type of Scenery: Parkland and water.
Condition of Pavement: Mostly paved; some hard-packed dirt.

The Bike Path:

This path runs from Ft. Point, located directly under the Golden Gate Bridge, to Aquatic Park, a swimming beach with a year-round water temperature of 55 degrees.

You might want to visit the historic fort before you start your ride. The red-brick fort, built in 1861 to protect the harbor, was obsolete by decade's end because of advancements in artillery. All the East Coast forts built in this style were destroyed during the Civil War so designers of the Golden Gate Bridge adapted the bridge itself in order to be able to keep this rare fort intact.

Riding east from the fort, you'll traverse the edge of the Presidio, a military base about to be transferred to the National Park Service. The Presidio's 1,400-acre preserve will soon provide miles of hiking and biking opportunities.

After the Presidio, you pass Crissy Field, a long and sandy beach. If you have the time, consider taking a short side trip to the Palace of Fine Arts and the Exploratorium, a participatory science museum begun by physicist Frank Oppenheimer.

You'll pass Marina Green, and most definitely will want to head out to the Wave Organ, a walk-in sculpture at the end of the long jetty near the Golden Gate Yacht Club where you can listen to the water of the bay as it plays on a series of pipes built into the amphitheater.

Next you'll pass Fort Mason and arrive at Aquatic Park, with its small swimming beach and cold salt water. Between Fort Mason and Aquatic Park you must ride up and over the somewhat steep hill at Black Point.

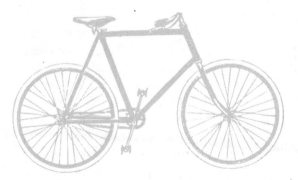

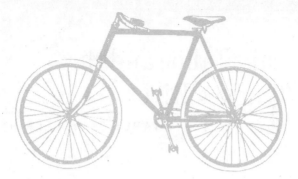

Food Facilities Nearby: Several restaurants along the water.

Restrooms: Ft. Point.

Special Precautions: You'll have to climb and descend Black Point.

Best Parking Lot: Ft. Point.

Directions: From Highway 1, get off at the last San Francisco exit, just before the Golden Gate Bridge. A sign will point to the toll plaza viewing area. At the first stop sign, turn right. At the second stop sign, turn left onto Lincoln Boulevard. Go about 3 blocks. Turn left onto the road leading to Ft. Point.

For More Information: Ft. Point National Historic Site, P.O. Box 29333, The Presidio, San Francisco, California 94129. Tel.: (415) 556-1693.

 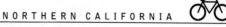

8. Lake Tahoe and the Truckee River

General Description:

17 miles of paved path running along the shore of Lake Tahoe and up the Truckee River.

Level of Difficulty: Average.

Type of Scenery: The crystal-blue water of Lake Tahoe with snow-covered peaks in the distance; the rippling mountain water flowing down the Truckee River; lots and lots and lots of traffic.

Condition of Pavement: Quite rough in places.

The Bike Path:

We had heard many good things about the Lake Tahoe bike path. We were disappointed. We hate to say so, but we felt that sections of the path that parallel Highway 89 were very dangerous. Highway 89 is a crowded main road along which motorists travel quite fast. The bike path travels alongside, crossing and recrossing many times, often without the help of a stoplight.

This is called a "Class 1" bike path, meaning that it's separated from the road. But it didn't seem safely separated to us. It often seemed like a "Class 2" bike lane, a striped bit of highway. If traffic doesn't bother you, this ride is fine, but we wouldn't bring children along.

If you ride here, you will enjoy the beauty of Lake Tahoe's shoreline. There are some sections that do manage to get away somewhat from the road, and you'll pass by many great parks and public beaches. The path ends at Sugar Pine Point State Park, a good place to swim. If you're comfortable locking your bike and walking, you'll find lots of places to do so along this path, but beware: this is major bike-theft territory.

The path we *did* love, an outstanding family ride, is the 5-mile section from Tahoe City up the Truckee River. This much safer path is somewhat distant from the highway. You'll ride along the cold and clear Truckee River, just a bit larger than a stream when it runs out of the lake. At the end of this path is a picnic area and a restaurant.

64 Acre Park, at the intersection of Highways 89 and 28, is a good central focal point for both the shoreline and the riverside paths. You can park in the large lot here and ride along the shoreline path, which extends more than 10 miles along the lake. When you've had enough, you can turn around and ride back to 64 Acre Park and set out along the riverside path.

For the Avid Cyclist: Tahoe is a major center for mountain biking. At many points along both of these paved paths, dirt trails spin off. There are many bike shops in the area which provide extensive information on the mountain-biking opportunities here.

Food Facilities Nearby: Tahoe City, and at the end of the Truckee River path.

Restrooms: At many points all along the way.

Special Precautions: The bike path along the Lake Tahoe shoreline is dangerous. Expect crowds. Expect problems with motor traffic on the highway.

This trail is snow-covered from early fall until May.

Best Parking Lot: 64 Acre Park.

Directions: From Interstate 80, take Highway 89 south to Tahoe City. When you reach the intersection with Highway 28, Highway 89 bends very sharply south along the lake. Look immediately for 64 Acre Park.

For More Information: Tahoe City Public Utility District, Parks and Recreation Department, P.O. Box 33, Tahoe City, California 96145. Tel.: (916) 583-3796.

9. The Westcliff Drive Pathway and Natural Bridges State Park

SANTA CRUZ, CALIFORNIA

General Description:

A 2.5-mile climb from the Santa Cruz boardwalk and wharf to the top of the seaside cliffs, ending at Natural Bridges State Park.

Level of Difficulty: Very challenging.

Type of Scenery: The Santa Cruz boardwalk with its dizzying roller coasters and the mile-long wharf extending into the bay; two state parks; the town's famous surfing beaches; the cliffs of Santa Cruz, with Monterey Bay below and the Pacific Ocean in the distance; at the top, a 65-acre state beach and park with a parking area that's a great place to watch the sun set.

Condition of Pavement: Rough in spots.

General Background:

In Santa Cruz, the streets belong to the bicycles. Few cities are as bike oriented as this university town. Most of the major city thoroughfares have bike lanes. A few connector roads are bikes-only routes, meant to help bicycle commuters avoid the more traffic-congested areas. Most city buses have bike racks. Several bridges have bike lanes.

If you want to park your car when you visit this city and rely only on your bike, you'll find it easy and fairly safe to do so. There are so many bikes on these city streets that drivers tend to be more aware of them and to grant them more respect on the roads.

The Bike Path:

In terms of scenic rides Westcliff Drive is a don't-miss path!

Cliffside Drive, a steep and narrow road with many turns, slithers up from the busy seaside boardwalk and wharf. The path starts near the Giant Dipper roller coaster built in 1924, another don't-miss ride—if you're a roller-coaster fan. If you want to explore the boardwalk, you'll have to walk your bike. Riding on the boardwalk is forbidden.

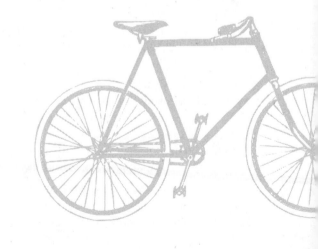

Nearby is the entrance to the municipal pier, a mile-long wharf said to be the longest wharf extending into the Pacific. It was built for the fishing fleets that once filled the bay and is now home to lots of trendy shops and a few really good restaurants. This wharf is busy. There's a two-lane road along here, so if you decide to ride your bike, beware. It's not going to be a peaceful, oceanside ride. You'll be combating car fumes, noise, and pedestrian congestion. There are plenty of places to lock your bike, but you also should be aware that bike theft is a major industry here.

The bike path up the cliffs begins at the corner of Beach and Washington Streets and follows the automobile road. It's easy to see why almost everybody in town makes it a habit to ride, jog, or walk up these heights in the early evening. You get a great workout *and* the reward of a fantastic sunset from the best vantage point in town.

Obviously built to accommodate the popularity of the cliffs, the bike path starts at the bottom as a very wide sidewalk, but as you ascend, the path becomes more independent of the road and the ride more dramatic.

First you'll come to Lighthouse Field State Beach, a 35-acre park owned by the state but managed by the city. You'll also ride past surfing beaches and a surfing museum. Even if you're not a surfer, we suggest visiting the museum. There's a whole American subculture here that's fascinating to learn about.

If you want to ride to the top of this path, you should be in good physical shape. The climb is steady and steep, but the view from the top is something you don't want to forgo.

For the Avid Cyclist: Some cyclists ride up the cliff path and through the roads in the state park. On the other side of the park, there are roads that lead to the campus of the University of California at Santa Cruz (another great bike path; see separate entry) and to Wilder Ranch State Park. Expect these roads to be crowded. The traffic will be moving quite quickly. Wilder Ranch has dirt trails for mountain cyclists.

Food Facilities Nearby: On the boardwalk.

Restrooms: On the boardwalk.

Special Precautions: No bike riding on the boardwalk.

This is a very steep path. If you are not in condition, plan to rest or to walk you bike frequently.

This is not a good path for children, unless they are particularly competent cyclists.

Best Parking Lot: Natural Bridges State Park; beach/boardwalk parking lot.

Directions: From Highway 1 (called Mission Street within city limits) turn west onto Bay Street. Follow Bay Street to the ocean. (There will be lots of signs.) To get to Natural Bridges State Park, turn right onto Westcliff Drive. At the end of the drive is the state park. To get to the boardwalk parking lot, turn left and follow the signs.

For More Information: City of Santa Cruz Parks and Recreation Department, 323 Church Street, Santa Cruz, California 95060. Tel.: (408) 429-3777.

10. The River Levee Bikeway

General Description:

A 4-mile flat path running along the east and west levees of the San Lorenzo River, crossing at the river's mouth on a railroad trestle.

Level of Difficulty: Very easy.

Type of Scenery: The Santa Cruz boardwalk-and-beach scene; urban environment; the river and tidal area of the Pacific Ocean; the railroad trestle.

Condition of Pavement: Rough in places.

The Bike Path:

This levee system of the San Lorenzo River has been paved to accommodate bicycle and pedestrian traffic. On the east levee the path is not contiguous. The path along the west levee is much more suited to recreational cycling.

The west-bank path extends along the river from its northernmost point at Josephine Street, just south of Highway 1, all the way to the boardwalk and railroad trestle.

At about the halfway point, a bike-and-pedestrian bridge leads across the river to San Lorenzo Park and some of the levee path along the river's east bank. San Lorenzo is a good place for a rest or picnic.

This is an interesting urban area. You can leave the

bike path and explore the city, either on foot or on bike. You'll find trendy stores, good restaurants, coffee shops, and great bookstores.

Farther south along the path, the boardwalk comes into view. You can walk your bike along the boardwalk, but you can't ride here. To get up to the railroad trestle look for the entrance ramp and a sign asking you to walk your bike.

Across the trestle is a wooden walkway up the river-bank to the street. You can ride up this walkway, but you'll have to ride on a very busy street when you get to the top. The bike path doesn't pick up again for several blocks. Traffic is fast, so stick to the sidewalk.

For the Avid Cyclist: For a nice out-and-back ride of about 10 miles, mostly on bike paths, start from Natural Bridges State Park (see separate entry). You'll ride down the cliffs, through Lighthouse Field State Beach, past the Steamer Lane surfing beach to Beach Street. The bike path ends here. You'll have to ride on Beach Street for several blocks until you pick up the River Levee path. Beach Street is one-way and has a wide, flat bike lane.

At the end of the street you'll see the railroad tres-tle in front of you and the west-bank river levee path to your left. Ride several miles up this levee to the bike-and-pedestrian bridge that crosses the river. Here you can either cross to San Lorenzo Park or turn left to the downtown area.

Return to Natural Bridges by the same route. Be sure to leave energy for the final uphill challenge.

Food Facilities Nearby: By the boardwalk.

Restrooms: Along the boardwalk.

Special Precautions: The east bank of the river levee has paved paths, but they are not always contiguous. You may find yourself contending with traffic at several points.

Best Parking Lot: The boardwalk area parking lot.

Directions: From Highway 1 (Mission Street) take Bay Street south to the beach. Turn left and follow signs for parking.

For More Information: City of Santa Cruz Parks and Recreation Department, 323 Church Street, Santa Cruz, California 95060. Tel.: (408) 429-3777.

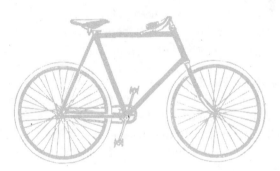

11. The University of California at Santa Cruz Bike Path

SANTA CRUZ, CALIFORNIA

General Description:

A short-but-sweet-but-hilly ride of 1.5 miles through the center of this college campus with some terrific views of Santa Cruz and the Pacific Ocean.

Level of Difficulty: Very challenging.
Type of Scenery: The university campus; coastal views.
Condition of Pavement: Good.

The Bike Path:

This path runs through the Great Meadow, an area filled with deer and posted with mountain-lion warnings. You'll get spectacular views of Monterey Bay, the Pacific Ocean, and the coastline from Santa Cruz all the way down to the city of Monterey.

But beware. The path from south to north is a grueling uphill climb, even for quite fit cyclists. And at beginning and end, the bike path feeds onto campus roads where you'll have to bike in among the cars. During weekdays, you'll also have to contend with buses that bring students from the city. If you're just beginning to ride, or have young children with you, you may not enjoy this path, despite its beauty.

But if you can cope with all these factors, you'll have a terrific time riding here. The university campus is set apart from the city, to the north and east of the urban center, on property that was formerly a ranch. Glenn Coolidge Drive runs along the southern edge of the campus. You can access the bike path as well as the campus roads from this drive.

The northern end of the path joins a system of roads that leads to most of the campus buildings.

Food Facilities Nearby: Campus snack bars.

Restrooms: Campus buildings open to the public.

Special Precautions: Steep terrain. Cyclists should be fit and skilled.

Best Parking Lot: The U.C. Santa Cruz campus.

Directions: From Highway 1, take the Bay Street exit. Go north. Cross High Street. Enter the campus area. This will be Glenn Coolidge Drive. The Carriage House will be on your right. The bike path will be on your left.

For More Information: The University of California at Santa Cruz, Bicycling Program Co-ordinator, 1156 High Street, Santa Cruz, California 95064. Tel.: (408) 459-5495.

12. Coyote Creek Parkway

General Description:

A 15-mile path through open meadows, farms, and fields, over small bridges that cross the creek, with very few road crossings.

Level of Difficulty: Average.

Type of Scenery: Farms and ranches in the creek valley; the Santa Cruz Mountains to the west; open space and hills to the east; fruit orchards, horses and sheep; a well-preserved riverbank habitat with plentiful birdlife and many small animals; a short stretch near roads, but mostly isolated from highway noise.

Condition of Pavement: Excellent in some places, somewhat rough in a few northern sections.

The Bike Path:

Bike path aficionados will definitely want to ride on this pretty country path. On a map, it appears to begin at Anderson Reservoir, but this isn't the case. The path's beginning is actually at Burnett Avenue.

You'll begin riding north on pavement, but very quickly the road will turn to gravel. This will last for only a half-mile, but you'll share the gravel section with cars driving to a model-plane park adjacent to the path. The traffic won't be heavy, but you might meet a few vehicles.

Most of the ride through the southern section is a relaxing and meditative meander through open fields and along Coyote Creek, a 60-mile watercourse that flows north into San Francisco Bay. You'll see hawks and turkey vultures soaring above, great blue heron fishing in the creek, and scrub jays, red-winged blackbirds, and song-birds sitting on the tall grasses in the many open fields. You'll also see lots of small critters and farm animals. People have reported fox, bobcat, and coyote.

Like the American River bikeway (see separate entry), there are long stretches when the cyclist neither sees nor hears the water. Since the designers didn't feel locked into providing a constant view of the water, the path can be playful and interesting. Sometimes it runs around the edge of a field in a wide semicircle so the cyclist can see approaching riders across the way. You'll ride under euca-lyptus and sycamore, with several bike-and-horse rest stops that have hitching posts and picnic tables. (Horses have their own separate dirt trail that crosses the paved path from time to time.)

Next, you'll ride through open fields and leave the creek for a while. You'll pass the Riverside Golf Course, Coyote Ranch, and Parkway Lakes, a series of creek-side ponds where fishing is available. At this point a short stretch runs along busy Monterey Highway, then the path becomes separate from the road again. You'll ride under Highway 101 and on to Coyote Hellyer County Park.

We like this path for children who have outgrown the

flat-trail stage but are not yet ready for road biking or mountain biking. There's a sense of adventure here, a sense of riding through a different environment, that kids will find exciting and challenging.

The beginning of this trail is the most rustic.

Food Facilities Nearby: None.

Restrooms: Burnett Avenue staging area; the radio-controlled model-airplane area; Parkway Lakes; Coyote Hellyer County Park.

Special Precautions: There are fewer trail users here than on other trails closer to urban areas. Ride with a friend.

Bring plenty of water.

Best Parking Lot: The Burnett Avenue staging area; Coyote Hellyer County Park.

Directions: To Burnett Avenue from Highway 101, take the Cochrane Road exit. Go west 0.8 mile. Turn right onto Monterey Highway (Highway 82). Go 1 mile. Turn right onto Burnett Avenue. Go 1 mile. There is a dirt parking lot. Cross the bike bridge to get to the beginning of the trail.

For More Information: County of Santa Clara Parks and Recreation Department, 298 Garden Hill Drive, Los Gatos, California 95030. Tel.: (408) 358-3741.

13. The Los Gatos Creek Streamside Trail

CAMPBELL AND LOS GATOS, SANTA CLARA COUNTY, CALIFORNIA

General Description:

A 14-mile path with gentle hills, following a creek and lakeshore to the Lexington Reservoir Dam.

Level of Difficulty: Average.

Type of Scenery: Semi-wild riparian habitat; small ponds with ducks; urban parks with tot lots; a kid-size small railroad.

Condition of Pavement: Rough in some places.

General Background:

Oak Meadows Park and Vasona Lake County Park are guaranteed to keep kids busy. There are picnic areas, ballfields, and shade trees and lots of kid-oriented activities, like the Billy Jones Wildcat Railroad that crosses Los Gatos Creek on a miniature wooden bridge. When that get boring, there's a carousel, several tot lots and playgrounds, fishing, a waterfront playground, horseshoe pits, and volleyball. Paddleboats and rowboats are available to rent.

The Bike Path:

Water is the dominant theme along this path, which hugs the creek for most of the distance. The creek is semi-natural, filled with islands covered with plant life and trees. Several bridges cross the water. We liked the ultra-modern bike-and-pedestrian bridge over Vasona Lake.

The ride begins at the Lexington Reservoir Dam and runs through the city of Los Gatos, through Vasona Lake County Park, through Los Gatos Creek County Park with its several small ponds, and then on to the Blackford School, north of the center of Campbell.

At times during the 14 miles you'll be riding above the water, while at other times you're right beside the creekbed. The path does wash out.

Expect to encounter high-speed in-line skaters, cyclists training for racing, joggers, and lots of walkers.

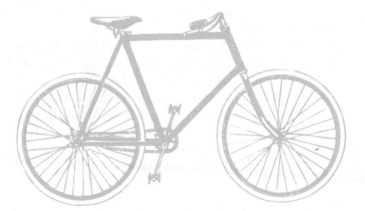

You'll have fun on this trail but you definitely won't be alone, even if you're out early in the morning.

There are a few hills. They are neither long nor forbidding, but because of the sharp bends you'll need to be careful not to run into people coming from the other direction.

Food Facilities Nearby: None.

Restrooms: Los Gatos Creek County Park; Vasona Lake County Park; Campbell Park.

Special Precautions: Be careful of other trail users. There are bound to be crowds here at almost any time during almost any day.

Best Parking Lot: Vasona Lake County Park.

Directions: From Highway 17, take the Highway 9 (Saratoga/Los Gatos Road) exit. Go east. Turn left onto Los Gatos Boulevard and left again onto Blossom Hill Road. The park will be on your right.

For More Information: County of Santa Clara Parks and Recreation Department, 298 Garden Hill Drive, Los Gatos, California 95030. Tel.: (408) 358-3741.

14. The Creek Trail at Alum Rock Park

General Description:

A 2.4-mile path, partially paved and partially hard-packed dirt, running up a canyon nicknamed "Little Yosemite."

Level of Difficulty: Average.

Type of Scenery: Big-leaf maple, white alder, and sycamore; honeysuckle vines, ferns, and wildflowers; lots of animal life.

Condition of Pavement: Some good pavement; some very rough pavement; some hard-packed dirt that may be ridden by a roadbike but will provide a very rough ride.

General Background:

In the middle of a sunny Sunday in this wild place, we watched a deer leap up from the creek, walk across the parking lot, and climb the canyon slopes. Snakes are common, as are rabbits, quail, turkey vultures, and red-tailed hawks. Park officials say there are bobcats. If you are a canyon connoisseur, Alum Rock belongs on your must-see list.

At Alum Rock Park, the oldest of California's parks,

you can ride through a semi-wild world, swim in the creek, soak in the aromatic mineral springs, and walk along ridges where you'll never hear the sounds of nearby San Jose, the state's second largest city. The canyon is nicknamed "Little Yosemite," a bit of an exaggeration, but understandable.

Alum Rock Canyon has nurtured humans since they first walked south from the Bering Strait. Native Americans liked the water, and when the Spanish walked north from Mexico, monks set up shop near here. The creek's name, Penetencia, refers to the baptisms performed in the aromatic water.

In the late nineteenth century, Alum Rock became fashionable. People traveled from San Francisco to sit in creekside tubs of smelly mineral water. There were 27 springs flowing with 7 different minerals. Visitors arriving on the Alum Rock Steam Railroad could use an indoor swimming pool filled with creek water or sit in a tea garden, restaurant, or plant pavilion. There were plans for residential hotels and "hospitals," but they came to naught.

The Bike Path:

We'd like to gloss over the state of the bike path because we want to convince you to visit the canyon, but, in good faith, we cannot. Only a small amount of this path, near the picnic area and the mineral bath/swimming area, is paved. The rest is dirt, and quite rough dirt at that. The trail begins as dirt at the Penetencia Creek Road park entrance and follows the bed of the old tourist railroad.

Following the railroad, you'll enjoy the sound of the creek for the whole ride. There's a canopy of trees above you and a ground cover of poison oak, an effective deterrent to straying from the beaten path. You'll cross a 120-foot-long railroad trestle, a popular photographic subject. At several points you can explore a variety of foot trails.

In the park's center are 14 acres of developed picnic and family facilities, including tot lots and restrooms with running water. Here you'll find the century-old stoneworks and ornate grottos where people soaked and swam and smelled the sulfuric waters, hoping for health. Several springs flow today with water pure enough for drinking.

The paved path runs through this area, then turns to dirt again. The canyon narrows. On this section, shared with walkers, you'll cross the stream on a small bridge. The path ends at a bridge with steps on both sides—obviously not a biking bridge. To travel on from here, you'll have to walk. The steep foot trail has many switchbacks, but if you walk up there you'll see the views that inspired the "Little Yosemite" sobriquet.

Food Facilities Nearby: None.

Restrooms: At the main visitor center; 7 outdoor restrooms along the way.

Special Precautions: Ride here with a friend; you are nearer than you think to the center of San Jose.

Best Parking Lot: The main visitor center.

Directions: From Highway 101, take the Alum Rock Avenue exit. Go east 4.5 miles. The road ends in the park.

For More Information: Alum Rock Park, 16240 Alum Rock Avenue, San Jose, California 95127-1307. Tel.: (408) 27-PARKS.

15. Nimitz Way and the East Bay Skyline National Recreation Trail

BERKELEY AND RICHMOND, CALIFORNIA, THE EAST BAY REGIONAL PARK DISTRICT

General Description:

A 4.1-mile segment of ridgeline that no cyclist or outdoor enthusiast will want to miss!

Level of Difficulty: Average.

Type of Scenery: Views, vistas, and views! From this ridge more than 1,000 feet above sea level, you'll see much of San Francisco Bay, the skyline of the central city, the Golden Gate Bridge, and the Pacific Ocean beyond; hundreds of acres of open parkland with ponds and reservoirs dotting the landscape; extensive groves of Monterey pine and eucalyptus; fields filled with wildflowers, springs, and tiny streams; riparian deciduous forests of alder, willow, bay laurel, and creek dogwood; lots of snakes, like gopher snakes, garter snakes, king snakes, and ringneck snakes, rubber boas, and western racers; many species of birds, including red-tailed hawk, Cooper's hawk, American kestrel, sharp-shinned hawk, and the ubiquitous turkey vulture.

Condition of Pavement: Excellent.

General Background:

Gold-rush frenzy permanently changed the color of the hills and ranchlands around the Bay Area. Where once there were brown hills dotted with green tufts of bunchgrass, after the gold rush there were hills covered with the pale greens of European grasses that burnt brown during the hotter seasons.

The European fortune-seekers brought cattle and sheep, and the hay to feed them. As the seed-filled hay spread around the countryside, the seeds flourished in the dry soils so like those of southern Europe. Soon the native bunchgrass disappeared.

As these European grasses spread like wildfire, they also *caused* wildfires. The bunchgrasses, separated by stretches of soil, were somewhat fire resistant, but the European grasses encouraged burning. As a result, cattle are a necessary environmental management tool in the Bay Area. Rather than destroying the environment as they do elsewhere, grazing cattle keep the hillside grasses short and fire resistant. Fire marshals tell landowners with tall grasses that they must plow up the grass or find cattle to eat it.

When you ride here, you'll share the fields with cattle, riding through gates and coasting over cattle guards. The cattle are protecting the native plants. About 80 percent of the species here are exotic imports from around the world. This 80 percent comprises only 70 percent of actual ground cover. Without cattle grazing, that 70 percent would quickly increase. The native grasses and wildflowers would disappear.

The Bike Path:

This 4-mile road once led to a NIKE missile site. Now it's one of the Bay Area's prime outdoor spots. The road has roller-coaster-like contours with pleasant, short climbs and quick drops. Around each bend you'll have a different perspective of the city below and the bay itself.

The path begins at Inspiration Point atop Wildcat Canyon Road. Nimitz Way begins with a fairly long, not-too-steep climb that curves around a hillside. On the other side, you'll get your first view of the city, the Golden Gate, and the Pacific.

Riding on, you'll enter a eucalyptus forest and breathe its chewing-gum aroma. Ecologists are divided over these trees. Some believe these Australian imports are giant weeds that overwhelm and destroy native plants. But others believe the trees promote birdlife and wildlife. Birds find the eucalyptus canopies to be havens of rest and isolation. Ground critters thrive in the deep flooring of leaves at each tree's base. Eucalyptus form extensive groves which are often thick enough to discourage humans from entering but allow other animals.

When you emerge from the eucalyptus, you'll ride through more cattle fields along the spine of these mountains. In several places gravel-covered fire roads branch off. You can follow these side spurs for more views of the city and the bay, but the deep gravel may be difficult to navigate.

For the Avid Cyclist: The pavement ends at a gate and a dirt/gravel road. Bikes may continue on this unmaintained road, but you will need fat tires and mountain-biking expertise.

This is a *very* popular mountain-biking area. Many fire roads are open to bikes, but others are expressly closed to them. For current information, check with the park.

To protect the newts, a section of the paved canyon road is closed to automobiles but open to bikes for a few weeks each year. Check with park officials for specific dates.

Food Facilities Nearby: None.

Restrooms: Inspiration Point parking lot.

Special Precautions: Nimitz Way is crowded on weekends and during the afternoon. If you hate crowds, go early.

Best Parking Lot: Inspiration Point.

Directions: From I-80 in Richmond, take the San Pablo Dam Road exit. Go east. Drive several miles. Wildcat Canyon Road will be on your right. At the top of this road with its many switchbacks will be Inspiration Point, with a large parking area.

For More Information: The East Bay Regional Park District, 2950 Peralta Oaks Court, P.O. Box 5381, Oakland, California 94605-0381. Tel.: (510) 562-PARK.

Wildcat Canyon Park Office, tel.: (510) 236-1262.

16. The Iron Horse Regional Trail

CONTRA COSTA COUNTY, CALIFORNIA, THE EAST BAY REGIONAL PARK DISTRICT

General Description:

A 15-mile, flat family recreation path that follows a former right-of-way for the Southern Pacific Railroad.

Level of Difficulty: Very easy.

Type of Scenery: The heart of the San Ramon Valley, with the hills of Mt. Diablo State Park to the north and the open space of Las Trampas Regional Wilderness to the south; suburban backyards and frequent shopping centers; local parks and community buildings; an intersection with the Contra Costa Canal Regional Trail; many road crossings.

Condition of Pavement: Excellent.

General Background:

Plans call for this trail, the backbone of Contra Costa County's extensive regional bikeways system, ultimately to extend from Suisun Bay north of Martinez to Pleasanton's Shadow Cliffs Regional Recreation Area, more than 30 miles distant. Officials believe much of the construction will be completed by 1998.

Along with the Contra Costa Canal Regional Trail (see

separate entry) the Iron Horse will provide a major bike route through the county. Several other important trails will connect to the Iron Horse soon: the Briones to Mt. Diablo Trail, the California Hiking and Riding Trail, the Las Trampas to Mr. Diablo Trail, and the Delta de Anza Regional Trail (see separate entry).

The Bike Path:

Beginning in San Ramon and ending in Walnut Creek, this urban trail follows Interstate 680 for much of its route, penetrating the heart of the congested valley and crossing many busy streets. It's a great way to commute from Walnut Creek to San Ramon. While motorists are stuck in traffic on I-680 or Danville Boulevard, you'll be whizzing along on the bike path, avoiding the honking horns.

This is a family trail, enthusiastically supported by its communities. It runs through residential areas and is flat and straight, with some very small hills near Walnut Creek. Near San Ramon, the path follows an irrigation canal through a fairly open area. You're bound to see Scouts and other children's groups, and local people out for an evening stroll, including members of a volunteer trail safety patrol. In-line skaters are welcomed. This popular and crowded path is not suitable for high speeds.

Food Facilities Nearby: Many good sandwich shops and restaurants in the frequent commercial areas en route.
Restrooms: San Ramon Community Park; Osage Park.
Special Precautions: Be careful of the many road crossings. Expect crowds after school and on weekends.
Best Parking Lot: San Ramon Community Park; many

informal, on-street parking opportunities all along the trail.

Directions: This trail parallels I-680. In Danville or San Ramon, you can take either the Sycamore Valley Road, the Crow Canyon Road, or the Bollinger Canyon exit. Head north on any of these roads for a very short distance, and you'll cross the path.

For More Information: The East Bay Regional Park District, 2950 Peralta Oaks Court, P.O. Box 5381, Oakland, California 94605-0381. Tel.: (510) 562-PARK.

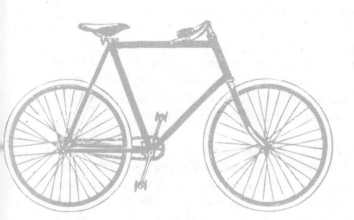

 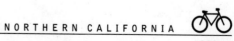

17. The Contra Costa Canal Regional Trail

CONCORD, PLEASANT HILL, PACHECO, AND WALNUT CREEK, CALIFORNIA, THE EAST BAY REGIONAL PARK DISTRICT

General Description:

A 14.2-mile canal-side path that's a major artery of the district's ambitious cross-county trail plan.

Level of Difficulty: Easy.

Type of Scenery: Very urban areas; lots of backyards; some open space with pleasant scenery; many road crossings, but several underpasses avoid the busiest highways.

Condition of Pavement: Rough in some spots.

General Background:

The East Bay Regional Park District and Contra Costa County are building a system of paved and unpaved paths that will almost rival its road system in complexity and completeness. When ready, cyclists will be able to ride almost anywhere in this huge county via the trail system.

The Contra Costa Canal and the Iron Horse (see separate entry) are the "interstate highways" of this transportation system, and they intersect in Walnut Creek. Most other trails will be accessible from one of these major routes.

The trail system already has more than 50 miles of pavement. When we asked how the district has achieved so much, we were told that the canal utility companies have been enthusiastically cooperative, allowing their canal-maintenance paths to double as bike-and-recreation paths. Couple that with the considerable amount of railroad right-of-way handed over to East Bay communities, and you have the makings of a world-class trail system.

Other canal companies have been frightened away from trail participation by their liability attorneys, but Contra Costa Water District, proud of its trail achievements, advertises the trail: the water district prints a special poster emphasizing its partnership in the trail-building process.

The Bike Path:

The Contra Costa Canal, more than 25 miles long, supplies water to many communities along its route. Beginning in Concord and ending in Walnut Creek, the recreation path accompanying the canal is richly varied and well maintained. Sometimes you'll ride along a flat, straight path level with the canal. At other times you'll enjoy small, undulating hills. Toward the eastern end you'll be riding through some small foothills with a tiny bit of elevation.

Be prepared for many road crossings. A few underpasses avoid major routes, such as I-689, but in general you're on your own at intersections.

Some segments of this trail are more pleasant than others. We found the city noise overwhelming near Walnut Hill. Our favorite segment was the ride through Pleasant Hill, where there were small, rolling hills and nice landscaping along the path, contributed by supportive neighbors.

One little scene belonged in *House Beautiful*: a 7-foot rosebush covered with pink blooms stood beside a pretty wooden footbridge leading from a private backyard to the path. We like these artistic touches that show the importance a neighborhood places on its recreation path. Landscaping a section of path as though it were a front yard sends a message: The path is valued as much as the road.

Food Facilities Nearby: Sandwich shops and restaurants at many intersections.

Restrooms: Heather Farm City Park.

Special Precautions: Ride with a friend; this is a busy city.

Best Parking Lot: Heather Farm City Park.

Directions: From I-680, take the Ygnacio Valley Road exit. Go east. Turn left onto San Carlos Drive and follow signs for Heather Farm.

For More Information: The East Bay Regional Park District, 2950 Peralta Oaks Court, P.O. Box 5381, Oakland, California 94605-0381. Tel.: (510) 562-PARK.

18. Coyote Hills Regional Park

NEWARK, CALIFORNIA, THE EAST BAY REGIONAL PARK DISTRICT

General Description:

A must-ride, 3.5-mile path, the "Pacific Coast Highway" of bike paths, leading to many miles of paths, paved and unpaved, through regional parkland and the National Wildlife Refuge.

Level of Difficulty: Average.

Type of Scenery: Golden-brown grasslands, red hills, and green marshes; tideland, salt ponds, and distant views across the bay; birdlife of every size and color, including the endangered California clapper, peregrine falcon, and California least tern; sky and water and peace and quiet.

Condition of Pavement: Excellent.

General Background:

According to the ancient Ohlone people, the entire San Francisco Bay is a pawprint made by a giant coyote. The Ohlone lived around the bay for 4,000 years and left more than 400 shell-and-debris mounds circling the bay. Most have been destroyed, but you can visit one of them, under the guidance of a naturalist, when you visit this regional park. Call ahead to arrange the tour.

These park hills are not related, geologically speaking,

to most East Bay hills. They are the remnants of a north-south mountain range long since worn away by erosion. These remaining rocky outcrops, pushed up from the ocean floor, are rust red and covered with tall grasses baked golden brown by the California sun. The vantage from atop these ancient hills is something you won't want to miss.

To the west, you'll see the open water of San Francisco Bay. To the south, you'll see the salt ponds, sloughs, and marshlands that create a healthy shore and clean bay. To the north, you'll see the channelized Alameda Creek and the 12-mile Alameda Creek Regional Trail (see separate entry).

And to the east, you'll see a marsh distinguished by its rich green color. This particular marsh—the Demonstration Urban Stormwater Treatment Marsh—shows what can be accomplished when people are determined to solve an environmental problem. The 55-acre research project purifies stormwater runoff, filtering it of heavy metals and hydrocarbons before it enters the bay.

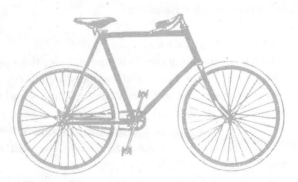

The Bike Path:

The bike path and park have all the right ingredients: water, hills, color, interest, sea breeze, natural beauty.

The loop circling this 1,000-acre island park (it essentially is an island, although the tide doesn't come up as high as it did a century ago) is fairly easy. Begin from the main parking lot and ride north on the path. You'll be riding above the marshland, circling the island on a bench road carved into the hillsides. You arrive quickly at the connection to the Alameda Creek Regional Trail (see separate entry).

Continuing along the loop trail, called the Bayview Trail, you'll ride above the bay and the National Wildlife Refuge, climbing and dipping with the roll of the hills, seeing spectacular views with each bend in the path.

At the Meadowlark Trail you'll see a paved road leading to the right. This is a very steep climb. We suggest you try it. At the top, you can see much of southern San Francisco Bay but you won't *hear* anything but birdsong and the wind in the grasses below.

For the Avid Cyclist: The Meadowlark Trail is a loop, but much of it is dirt. Cyclists may ride the dirt trails, as well as many others that crisscross the park and refuge. Near the Meadowlark Trail, the No Name Trail leads to the Shoreline Trail and the Apay Way Trail leads to the National Wildlife Refuge Visitor Center. A few of these park trails are closed to biking; check on trail status at a visitor center to be sure.

Many of these park trails are accessible to road bikes or to hybrid bikes and are technically fairly easy to ride. Some of them lead out across the levee system, a flat expanse that's fun to explore and easy for beginners. If you have any interest in dirt-trail riding, this is a good place to try the sport out.

Food Facilities Nearby: None.

Restrooms: Visitor center and parking area.

Special Precautions: This is a wildlife sanctuary. Officials ask you to bike only on trails where bikes are specifically invited.

Best Parking Lot: Visitor center.

Directions: From Interstate 880, take the Highway 84 exit. Turn right onto Ardenwood Boulevard. Turn left onto Commerce Drive. This becomes Patterson Ranch Road and leads to the park.

For More Information: The East Bay Regional Park District, 2950 Peralta Oaks Court, P.O. Box 5381, Oakland, California 94605-0381. Tel.: (510) 562-PARK.

Coyote Hills Regional Park Visitor Center, Tel.: (510) 795-9385.

San Francisco Bay National Wildlife Refuge Visitor Center and Headquarters, Tel.: (510) 792-0222.

19. The Alameda Creek Regional Trail

UNION CITY AND ALVARADO, CALIFORNIA, THE EAST BAY REGIONAL PARK DISTRICT

General Description:

A 12-mile flat path along a major, channelized creek lined with riprap.

Level of Difficulty: Very easy.

Type of Scenery: A wide creekbed with several large, dammed ponds toward the path's eastern end; San Francisco Bay with miles of levees and salt ponds at the western end; several underpasses, *no* road crossings; picnic sites and fishing ponds; several parks; suburban backyards; a short stretch near a busy road.

Condition of Pavement: Good.

General Background:

Alameda Creek, the largest of Alameda County's flowing streams, once teemed with spawning salmon. The Ohlone people fished and hunted here, and Kit Carson trapped the creek's beaver. But farming and later industrialization changed the character of the creek. Now its banks are locked in place with stone riprap. Toward its mouth, the creek is almost dry much of the year; the section below Niles Canyon has been dammed to make ponds.

The best thing that's happened recently to the creek is the recreation path that runs for 12 miles along both the north and south banks. On the north bank, the soft surface is designed for horses as well as hikers. On the south bank, the pavement accommodates bicycles.

The Bike Path:

This flat ride runs from Niles Canyon, where the creek emerges from the hills, to the bay. Much of the ride is along the open bank, with frequent stands of eucalyptus and other shade trees. There are lots of picnic tables and rest areas along the route.

The path begins at Vallejo Mill Historic Park. The creek here is not channelized and water access is easy. Starting down the path you'll pass several small dams and ride under several automobile bridges that cross the water. Below this segment, the water is intermittent. You'll pass apartment houses and neighborhood developments, as well as a few horse farms.

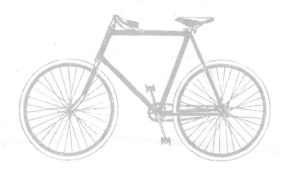

Several staging areas have groves of shade trees, drinking water, and picnic tables. The ride is serene and quite pleasant. Your only encounter with automobiles will be one brief stretch when the path nears busy Paseo Padre Parkway. Otherwise, although you're in a very built-up area, you'll hardly hear the cars. This is a good ride for someone interested in some quiet time for meditation.

At the western end of the path, 11 miles from Vallejo Mill, is Coyote Hills Regional Park (see separate entry).

For the Avid Cyclist: We suggest combining the Alameda Creek Trail with the loop around Coyote Hills Regional Park. Begin at Vallejo Mill Historic Park and ride west almost to the end of the paved trail. On your left you'll see a short paved side spur leading up into the Coyote Hills. Signposts mark this spot. You can ride around the hills, explore some side spurs, and return to your starting point at the east end of the Alameda Creek Trail to complete a ride of almost 30 miles without one road crossing.

To add even more miles, explore dirt roads and easy dirt trails in Coyote Hills. You can also add to this ride by heading south out of the regional park and entering the National Wildlife Refuge on the Apay Way Trail. There are enough dirt roads and dirt trails in this area to keep you busy for a very long day. They are more challenging than the flat pavement of the Alameda Trail, but they are fairly easy.

Food Facilities Nearby: None.

Restrooms: Niles Canyon staging area; Shinn Pond; Isherwood staging area; Robert Cann Park; Beard staging

area; Coyote Hills Regional Park Visitor Center;
National Wildlife Refuge Visitor Center and Headquarters.

Special Precautions: The Alameda Creek Trail is paved on
the south side and unpaved on the north side. At various points along the trail, you may cross from the
paved to the unpaved side on automobile bridges. If
you want to get from the unpaved path to Coyote Hills
and the National Wildlife Refuge, you'll have to cross
far upstream. There is no bridge near that end of the
trail.

Best Parking Lot: Niles staging area of Vallejo Mill Historic
Park.

Directions: From Highway 880, take the Highway
84/Decoto Road exit. Go north. Turn right onto Niles
Boulevard. Cross Mission Boulevard. At the fork of
Niles Canyon Road and Old Canyon Road, look for
the staging area and the path.

For More Information: The East Bay Regional Park District,
2950 Peralta Oaks Court, P.O. Box 5381, Oakland,
California 94605-0381. Tel.: (510) 562-PARK.

20. The Lafayette/Moraga Trail

**LAFAYETTE AND MORAGA, CALIFORNIA,
THE EAST BAY REGIONAL PARK DISTRICT**

General Description:

A very pretty 7.75-mile suburban path, with hills and bends to add to the fun of this short-but-sweet ride.

Level of Difficulty: Average.

Type of Scenery: Las Trampas Creek and Bollinger Canyon; well-cared-for suburban homes; a recreation-path-friendly population has landscaped sections of the path; several large parks and open areas; a short section along a busy road; a short ride along sidewalks through a commercial center.

Condition of Pavement: Mostly good; rough in a few places. Difficult to follow for several blocks southwest of Moraga Commons.

General Background:

Several years ago, a university professor wanted to know how residents felt about their recreation trail after it had been around for a while. The Lafayette-Moraga Trail was one of the three he studied. He found that nearly all the residents interviewed found the trail an asset to the neighborhood. Some claimed the trail increased their property values. Many who admitted to opposing the trail at first said they now recognized its value and used it frequently.

Since we knew this trail enjoyed the loyalty of the neighborhood, we weren't that surprised to find the Lafayette/Moraga Trail treated like a main street in the neighborhood. Homeowners landscape their path frontage with elegance. "For Sale" signs are hung along the path and neighbors gather to walk and talk here in the evenings.

The pride of the residents is reflected in the fun of the ride. We had a good time and, although we didn't ride past any spectacular sights, there are pretty gardens and spring wildflowers. You'll ride through parks and greenbelts with pleasant views of soft hills. And although you'll encounter people on the trail, you probably won't encounter excessive crowds.

The Bike Path:

Just seeing what's around the corner on this ride will keep you from suffering the boredom typical of some suburban bike paths. The trail begins at the Olympic staging area on the Pleasant Hill Road near Highway 24. It ends at the Valle Vista staging area on Canyon Road in Moraga, near Redwood Regional Park. If you plan to bike the length of the path and back, we suggest you begin at the Olympic staging area.

The first half of the trail is a very gentle but quite persistent uphill ride. For the first few miles, you'll be riding near Las Trampas Creek, but you'll see it only intermittently. You'll pass residential areas with pleasant gardens and yards. Prepare for some kidney-rattling rides across several wooden bridges made with old railroad ties.

About the time you reach the crest of this gentle climb, you'll also reach open space. For much of the ride, we're sorry to say, you'll follow St. Mary's Road, a two-lane road with noisy traffic. When you enter the open area, the road stays behind. This section is much quieter and conducive to peaceful enjoyment of the natural surroundings.

You'll begin to ride downhill now, encountering a few slopes of 5–7 degrees. They're short. Enjoy the coast down; they won't be *that* difficult on the return trip. You'll ride down into Moraga Commons and then into a commercial district.

We lost the path here for a few moments. It becomes a sidewalk that leads to a major intersection so you must cross the street and continue along the sidewalk. There are small, unobtrusive brown wooden posts with discreet white arrows that will point you in the correct direction. They'll guide you for the next few blocks until the pavement of the bike path splits off from the road again.

Don't give up and turn back. The short bit of remaining trail is worth the effort. Initially, you'll enter what might best be described as "suburban backcountry" behind some houses and through some odd little side streets and alleyways. When you come to EBMUD/Redwood Regional Park, you'll ride up a few hills with some steep climbs. There are some nice views from here until the trail's end.

We liked the ride back because of the final long downhill coast. It's not steep enough that you can coast all the way from the midway point to the Olympic staging area, but you'll definitely notice you're going downhill.

Food Facilities Nearby: None.

Restrooms: None.

Special Precautions: Watch for the brown trail signposts in the commercial section.

Best Parking Lot: Pleasant Hill Road.

Directions: From Highway 24, take Pleasant Hill Road south. Turn right onto Olympic Boulevard. Look for the staging area.

For More Information: The East Bay Regional Park District, 2950 Peralta Oaks Court, P.O. Box 5381, Oakland, California 94605-0381. Tel.: (510) 562-PARK.

21. The Delta de Anza Regional Trail

General Description:

A 4.6-mile, flat path that follows the Contra Costa Canal and a utility corridor through the county's northeastern corner, near the Sacramento/San Joaquin River Delta.

Level of Difficulty: Very easy.

Type of Scenery: Suburban homes; busy roads; a small neighborhood park and a county park with reservoir; some meadows and open space.

Condition of Pavement: Rough in some places.

General Background:

This trail will eventually connect with the Contra Costa Canal Regional Trail (see separate entry), allowing cyclists to ride on paved paths all the way from the Contra Loma Regional Park into Walnut Creek. At Walnut Creek, you can turn onto the Iron Horse Regional Trail (see separate entry) and ride all the way down to San Ramon.

Ultimately, the Delta de Anza Regional Trail may extend more than 20 miles. For now, though, this remains a suburban path that gets lots of local family use.

The Bike Path:

This is a pleasant family-outing path, but be careful of the road crossings. Traffic travels here at high speeds. For a short while, the path runs parallel to busy James Donlon Boulevard.

The path touches the borders of two parks. Antioch Community Park is a pleasant park with paved side spurs, mowed grasslands, ball fields, and a much-used tot lot. A paved path runs up a steep hill at the far west end of the parking lot. This takes you through parkland to the Contra Loma Regional Park, with its 80-acre reservoir and swimming beach. You can rent kayaks, sailboards, and pedal boats during the summer.

Adjacent to Contra Loma is the Black Diamond Mines Regional Preserve. Coal was mined here for several decades. This preserve of nearly 4,000 acres has interesting interpretive programs, but biking is not permitted.

Food Facilities Nearby: None.

Restrooms: Antioch Community Park; Contra Loma Regional Park.

Special Precautions: This trail requires crossing several busy roads without the help of either a bike-and-pedestrian bridge or traffic lights.

Best Parking Lot: Antioch Community Park.

Directions: Take Highway 4 to the city of Antioch. Exit onto Contra Loma Boulevard. Go south 1.3 miles. Turn left (east) onto James Donlon Boulevard. The Antioch Community Park is on the right.

For More Information: The East Bay Regional Park District, 2950 Peralta Oak Court, P.O. Box 5381, Oakland, California 94605-0381. Tel.: (510) 562-PARK.

22. The Monterey Peninsula Recreation Trail

PACIFIC GROVE, MONTEREY, AND SEASIDE, CALIFORNIA

General Description:

A 4.8-mile path running through Monterey's restored waterfront area and along the high cliffs overlooking Monterey Bay, the nation's largest marine sanctuary. Everyone loves this ride!

Level of Difficulty: Very easy.

Type of Scenery: The restless waters of Monterey Bay, filled with wildlife like gray whales and California sea lions; the remarkable Monterey Bay Aquarium; beautifully maintained Victorian homes; musicians playing on street corners; John Steinbeck's Cannery Row; Fisherman's Wharf; Monterey State Beach.

Condition of Pavement: Excellent.

General Background:

Plans for this path were first conceived by the Monterey Peninsula Regional Park District and other governmental agencies in 1978. When the project was completed a decade later, the 5-mile trail had cost more than $7 million.

By 1998, the Monterey trail will connect to the Fort Ord Trail (see separate entry), by way of a to-be-constructed segment through Sand City. When this happens, you'll be able to ride along the coast on bike paths all the way from Pacific Grove north to Marina, a distance of about 12 miles.

The Bike Path:

Running from Lover's Point in Pacific Grove to Canyon del Rey in Seaside, the trail includes history, natural beauty, and city-life excitement, all in 5 short miles. From Lover's Point, you'll ride a gentle downhill grade for the first mile or so. To your right, higher up on the cliffs, sit the century-old Victorian mansions owned by the elite when the city was the world's sardine-canning center.

To your left, 20 feet below, the waves splash against the granite outcroppings. You can stop along the way and rest beneath the cypress trees edging the cliffs above the water. Binoculars will serve you well here. In the distance you may see gray whales; nearby you'll find kayakers paddling the marine sanctuary kelp forests.

When you're ready to move on, the path leads into the cacophony of the urban center. Tourists are everywhere. Pedaled surreys, the kind with the fringe on top, clog the recreation path. There are walkers, roller-bladers, and loose dogs. On one street corner musicians are playing South American wooden flutes. On the next, drummers fill the street-corner space.

Colorful flower gardens and voluptuous shrubbery brighten the city walls. Stores open onto the path with welcoming signs, and there are cafes where people can eat with their skates on or their bikes nearby. This recreation path is an important commercial street, like Main Street used to be before automobiles depersonalized downtown life.

Next, the path runs past Cannery Row, near Fisherman's Wharf and past the Maritime Museum. Following the route is a bit dicey here. You'll have to negotiate a parking lot, ride past the Maritime Museum, and ride next to an automobile tunnel.

Crossing Figueroa Street, you're rewarded for your persistence. This segment runs by the barrier dunes of the state beach, where there are bike racks. You can climb the steep wooden stairs to the top of the dunes and enjoy the water on the other side. Beyond the state beach is a stand of eucalyptus trees and a windsurfing beach where you can watch the action.

The path currently ends in Seaside, at Canyon del Rey. To ride farther, you have two bike-path options. You can turn right onto Canyon del Rey and ride a half-block to Laguna Grande Regional Park (see separate entry), where there is a short and easy path around some freshwater, or you can ride 1.5 miles on-street along Del Monte Boulevard to pick up a 4-mile path, the Fort Ord Trail (see separate entry). Sand City is building a bike-path connector to eliminate this on-street ride. The completion date is uncertain.

For the Avid Cyclist: At the westerly end of this recreation trail in Pacific Grove, some cyclists continue riding along the shoreline on the automobile roads. You'll ride on Oceanview Avenue and Sunset Drive, around the perimeter of the peninsula, past Point Pinos and Asilomar State Beach to Pebble Beach.

You'll see some rugged and beautiful seashore, but you must be able to contend with heavy traffic and a very narrow, twisting road. These roads are hilly and challenging. In places, the striped bike lanes are quite narrow and even disappear completely. Many cyclists ride these roads, but we don't recommend them for children or for adults who dislike traffic.

Food Facilities Nearby: Many in the center of Monterey.

Restrooms: None.

Special Precautions: None.

Best Parking Lot: Laguna Grande Regional Park.

Directions: From Highway 1, turn onto the road called Canyon del Rey. Go in the direction *away* from the water, about a half-block. Look for the regional park and parking lot.

For More Information: The City of Monterey Recreation Department, Monterey City Hall, Pacific and Madison, Monterey, California 93940. Tel.: (408) 646-3866.

Pacific Grove Recreation Department, 300 Forest Avenue, Pacific Grove, California, 93950. Tel.: (408) 648-3130.

The Monterey Peninsula Regional Park District, P.O. Box 935, Carmel Valley, California 93924. Tel.: (408) 659-4488.

23. Laguna Grande Regional Park

General Description:

A 1-mile path circling the park lagoon, only a short distance from the current eastern end of the Monterey Peninsula Recreation Trail.

Level of Difficulty: Very easy.
Type of Scenery: Parkland and water.
Condition of Pavement: Good.

The Bike Path:

This regional park of 35 acres has a 12-acre freshwater lagoon encircled by a flat and easy paved bike path. You'll find lots of ducks and other waterfowl here, and some lush freshwater foliage. The park has picnic facilities and playgrounds for children. No swimming is allowed in the water.

We suggest it as a nice addition to the Monterey Peninsula Recreation Trail (see separate entry). You can ride from Lover's Point to the path's eastern end at Canyon del Rey, turn right on Canyon del Rey, and ride only a half-block (riding on the sidewalk is permitted here) to the park entrance.

The park makes a nice halfway resting point. Ride

around the lagoon path, have a picnic lunch, and then head back down the Monterey path, from whence you came.

Food Facilities Nearby: None.

Restrooms: Yes.

Special Precautions: If you make the connection from Monterey to Laguna Grande along Canyon del Rey, be aware that this is neither a bike path nor a bike lane. You are legally permitted here to ride on the sidewalk, if you prefer.

Best Parking Lot: Laguna Grande Regional Park.

Directions: From Highway 1, turn onto the road called Canyon del Rey, heading *away* from the salt water. Go a half-block. Look for the park.

For More Information: The Monterey Peninsula Regional Park District, P.O. Box 935, Carmel Valley, California 93924. Tel.: (408) 659-4488.

24. The Fort Ord Trail

General Description:

A 4-mile path through the Highway 1 right-of-way; soon to be transformed into a beautiful seashore path through a new state beach.

Level of Difficulty: Challenging.

Type of Scenery: The Fort Ord Reservation; miles of dunes and shoreline; a four-lane highway; replanting of local vegetation.

Condition of Pavement: Poor in places; reconstruction is scheduled.

General Background:

Currently, 4 miles of paved bike path extend through this highway right-of-way, sometimes coming quite close to Highway 1. In its current state, we wouldn't recommend this path as a recreation ride for casual cyclists, although it is used as a training route by competitive cyclists.

However, this is changing. The shoreline between Sand City and Marina, the former military property known as Fort Ord, is being turned into a state beach, a task expected to take several years. A few sections of the park will open by 1997 or 1998.

When this is done, a new 4-mile path running along

the oceanfront will be built to complement the path already existing parallel to Highway 1.

If it goes well, sometime after the end of the decade, you'll be able to ride along the seashore on bike paths for 12 miles, from Lover's Point in Pacific Grove, the westerly end of the Monterey Peninsula Recreation Trail (see separate entry), through Monterey, Seaside, and Sand City to end in Marina.

The Bike Path:

This bike path, as it currently exists, closely parallels Highway 1. Several precarious segments bring the cyclist almost directly alongside very heavy, high-speed traffic. This is not a good place for kids, or for adults who dislike traffic.

The bike path was built in the late 1960s and early 1970s. Since so much of the current situation is open to change, we suggest you contact the agency listed below to find out how far construction has progressed.

Currently, the path begins at Ord Terrace, near the intersection of Highway 1 and Del Monte Road, and runs north along the highway. The path crosses Locke Paddon Park, a wetlands area with picnic facilities, and ends at Reservation Road in Marina.

Food Facilities Nearby: None.

Restrooms: None.

Special Precautions: You'll be riding extremely close to high-speed traffic. You must be a competent cyclist.

Best Parking Lot: Parking is currently catch-as-catch-can.

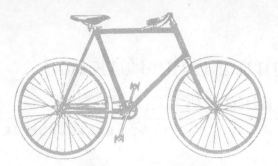

Directions: To pick up the southern end of the trail as it currently exists, take Highway 1. Exit at Del Monte Boulevard and look for Ord Terrace.

For More Information: The Monterey Peninsula Regional Park District, P.O. Box 935, Carmel Valley, California 93924. Tel.: (408) 659-4488.

 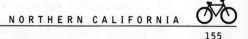

25. Spring Lake Park and Annadel State Park

SANTA ROSA, CALIFORNIA

General Description:

A 3.5-mile paved path that winds through hilly parkland, around a large lake, and alongside a man-made lagoon with a public swimming area.

Level of Difficulty: Easy.

Type of Scenery: Canopies of native trees; wild tangles of vines and moss hanging from branches of native oak; ponds and wetlands and vernal pools; picnic areas and camping areas.

Condition of Pavement: Good.

General Background:

Santa Rosa is the commercial center of the Sonoma Valley. Compared with neighboring Napa Valley, Sonoma is downscale, a fact which some Sonomans consider a blessing.

Despite that fact, Santa Rosa is a far-from-rural city. It is the home of the Ripley Memorial Museum as well as the Luther Burbank Home and Gardens, where you can see, among other things, the horticulturist's greenhouse and 4-acre laboratory-garden.

The city also hosts some memorable traffic jams. But if

you want to escape the wine-country hubbub and enjoy a serene ride through parklands where you can barely hear a horn honk, you'll find 5,000 acres of public parks only a few minutes from Highway 12. There are three public parks—first city, then county, then state—all in a row. These parks offer a variety of cycling options, ranging from an easy ride around a lake to rides over unpaved, challenging terrain.

The Bike Path:

This is an excellent place for families. If you have a group with varying cycling interests and abilities, this is the place for you. Some of your cyclists can enjoy the flat lakeside path, while others can explore dirt roads or difficult trails. These are all within park confines, so you needn't worry about traffic.

If you begin at the county park staging area, you'll find a 2-mile paved path that circles Spring Lake. Most of this ride is quite flat, although you will encounter some mild, interesting hills around the northwestern shore.

If you continue along the path, you'll come to several picturesque knolls covered with wild tangles of vines and small oak trees. Farther on, you'll come to a picnic area, a boat launch, and, finally, a swimming lagoon open during the summer months.

Directly to the west of Spring Lake, near a small wetlands area, a paved path branches off to the west. This path heads to Lake Ralphine and the athletic fields at the other end of the city park. This path is much steeper; if you take it, expect quite a climb on your return trip.

If these paved paths are too easy or too short for you,

the parks are filled with compacted side trails open to cyclists. Many of these do not require mountain bikes, and are easy enough for most cyclists.

To the east of the county park, you'll have access to Annadel State Park, a 5,000-acre mostly undeveloped area which was once a major quarry for the cobblestone that paved the streets of San Francisco. The park does not have paved paths. It *does* have many dirt roads, fire roads, and dirt trails on which cyclists are permitted. The park also has lovely stands of redwoods, Douglas fir, and oaks.

Food Facilities Nearby: None. Picnic facilities are plentiful.

Restrooms: At the staging/parking areas for each of the three parks, open in season.

Special Precautions: The pavement around some sections of Spring Lake may wash out during heavy rains.

Best Parking Lot: Spring Lake Park (unless you plan to ride mostly on the dirt roads and trails of the state park).

Directions: From Highway 12, just east of the central area of Santa Rosa, take the Los Alamos Road exit. Head southwest. Cross Melita Road and turn right onto Montgomery Drive. You'll see the signs for the county park.

For More Information: Sonoma County Regional Parks, 2300 County Center Drive, Room 120A, Santa Rosa, California 95403. Tel.: (707) 527-2041.

26. Yosemite Valley Ride

YOSEMITE NATIONAL PARK, CALIFORNIA

General Description:

About 8 miles of mostly flat paths winding past Yosemite Valley's most popular sites.

Level of Difficulty: Easy.

Type of Scenery: Half Dome and Mirror Lake; Yosemite Falls; the wild and scenic Merced River; Yosemite Village, with its museums, gardens, and the Ansel Adams Gallery; the Awanee Meadow, North Dome, and the Royal Arch Cascade; Happy Isles Nature Center and the foot trail to Vernal Fall and Nevada Fall.

Condition of Pavement: Good.

General Background:

More than 4 million people visit Yosemite each year. Most come by car, get stuck in traffic jams, and end up seeing much of Yosemite's beauty from the perspective of a car window. They miss the sounds of birdsong, windsong, and flowing water.

On the bike path, riding through stands of ponderosa pine and incense cedar, you'll have a different experience. At the same time, you'll help protect this delicate natural resource. As in Utah's Zion National Park (see separate entry), automobile pollution is ruining the vegetation and water. In fact, if the shuttle experiment in Zion is successful, something similar may be implemented in Yosemite.

The Bike Path:

This bike path consists of a west loop and an east loop, connected by a short segment. The paths are generally separated from the busy automobile road, but several sections do parallel the automobiles. There are several road crossings and several segments where you must share the path with shuttle buses and service vehicles.

If you begin riding from Yosemite Lodge, you'll be near Yosemite Falls, 2,425 feet high, the tallest waterfall in Yosemite and the third-tallest in the world. Heading west, you'll ride through a large meadow and over the Merced River on a bike-and-pedestrian bridge made of heavy wooden timbers.

When the path curves back east along Southside Drive, a one-way automobile road, you'll see another open meadow fringed with cottonwoods and Yosemite Chapel. Built in 1879, this is the valley's oldest continually used building. Above the chapel, over a ridge, you'll see Half Dome rising straight up for a vertical mile, Yosemite's most easily recognizable symbol.

Along the path there are lots of exotic trees, imports brought by settlers a century ago—fruit trees, elm, and a sugar maple that turns fire-engine red in the fall, which was planted by photographer J. T. Boysen as a reminder of his New England home.

Next the path curves north, heading toward Yosemite Falls where you began. You'll cross the Merced River on another bike bridge and come to a "T" intersection. Turn right on the path and head toward Yosemite Village, the valley's business center with stores, restaurants, a visitor center, restrooms, and more.

Then you'll ride parallel to the automobile road for a mile to the other loop. This loop will take you through Curry Village and past several camping areas on a full-width road open to park vehicles. You'll arrive at Happy Isles Nature Center, where you'll want to lock your bike and walk along the Mist Trail to a set of waterfalls. Expect to get wet, even on the walk up to the falls.

You'll also pass the horseback riding stables (rides for the public range in length from several hours to several days; reserve well in advance), Mirror Lake, and Half Dome.

Single-speed bikes may be rented either at Curry Village, near the day-use parking lot, or at Yosemite Lodge.

Food Facilities Nearby: Several restaurants and snack opportunities at Yosemite Village.

Restrooms: Many restrooms throughout the valley.

Special Precautions: The bike paths are shared with park vehicles.

Best Parking Lot: Curry Village day-use parking.

Directions: Drive into the valley along the Southside Drive, a one-way road that enters the valley. Follow signs for Curry Village and for day-use parking.

For More Information: The U.S. Department of the Interior, National Park Service, P.O. Box 577, Yosemite, California 95389. Tel.: (209) 372-0200.

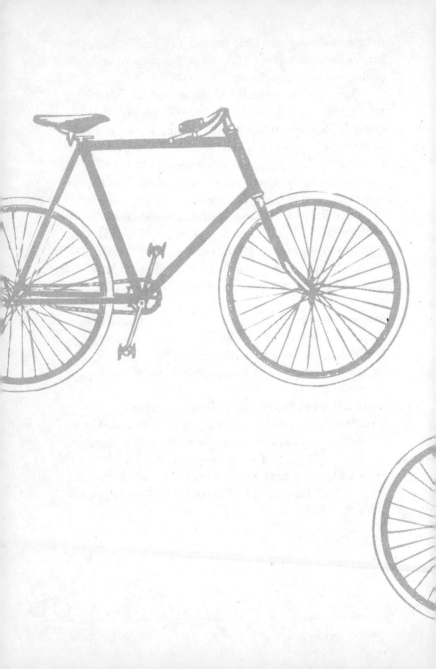

Southern
California

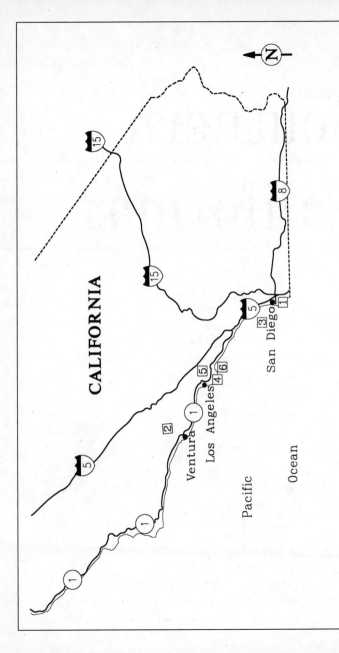

Southern California

1. The Silver Strand Bikeway

CORONADO AND IMPERIAL BEACH, CALIFORNIA

General Description:

About 10 miles of path following the shoreline of elegant Coronado and the Silver Strand.

Level of Difficulty: Very easy.

Type of Scenery: Salt water and sand; San Diego Bay and the city of San Diego across the water; the famous Hotel del Coronado, where presidents stay; several state and city public beaches and parks; a short on-street section.

Condition of Pavement: Good.

General Background:

When railroad tycoon Elisha Babcock and H. L. Story (of Story & Clark upright pianos—every school had one) came to this island in the 1880s, they recognized the obvious: this was the perfect elite resort destination. Story bought 4,100 acres of land for $110,000, Babcock joined him, and they began building. When the Hotel del Coronado opened in 1888, it was unlike anything ever seen on the California coast.

Today, with its eerie Victorian turrets, cupolas, and flying pennants, the hotel remains a city landmark. There are, by now, several other resorts in the area, as well as a slew of hotels and inns suited to the average pocketbook. The Silver Strand Bikeway takes you past the three most upscale of these resorts, where, guest or not, you're invited to walk the grounds.

Bring bike locks. There are many places where you'll want to walk through buildings and gardens.

The Bike Path:

To get to this well-known bike path from San Diego, many people ride the San Diego Bay Ferry, a 15-minute trip. You'll disembark at Ferry Landing Marketplace, a restaurant-and-boutique area, and follow a sidewalk for 2 blocks through the market area to get to the path. It's easy to find; just follow the flow of cyclists and skaters.

Across the water you'll see views of the San Diego skyline, with high-rise office buildings and city-center elegance. In the late afternoon, when the sun is low, you'll see an explosion of light and color as the sun reflects against the tinted glass windows of downtown.

Next comes Le Meridien, one of the three resorts and known for its aviaries and botanical gardens. There is also a migratory pond for birds that appears to be shared with the local duck population.

Past Le Meridien is Tidelands Park with a bayside beach where you can swim in the quiet bay waters. There is no lifeguard. You'll catch some good views of south San Diego Bay and the Navy ships in dock, then ride underneath the San Diego–Coronado Bay Bridge, a 2.3-mile-long sky-blue concrete creation that's equal to the Golden Gate in engineering majesty. When you pass the Coronado Municipal Golf Course, you'll turn left onto Glorietta

Boulevard and ride for more than a mile on this street in the company of lots of other cyclists and skaters.

When Glorietta Boulevard intersects 10th Street at the tennis courts, the separated bike path begins again. You'll see a yacht club, the Coronado Chart House, and the Hotel del Coronado across Orange Avenue. As at Le Meridien, you may tour the grounds and take a gander at this national historic landmark.

After the Hotel del Coronado, the path runs down the Silver Strand, the narrow 9-mile strip of sand protecting San Diego from the ravages of the Pacific Ocean. You'll pass Glorietta Bay Park, a small park with swimming facilities, water fountains, and play areas, then ride next to the Navy Amphibious Base, home of the Navy Seals, where you are definitely *not* invited to stroll.

You'll pass a beach reserved for the endangered least terns, then come to the Loews Coronado Bay Resort, with several cafes open to the public. Next comes the Silver Strand State Beach, with public swimming areas, and then Coronado Cays, an exclusive residential area. The bike path ends at Palm Avenue in Imperial Beach.

Along the Silver Strand this path parallels Highway 75, a major four-lane highway. You'll be separated enough to be safe, but you won't escape the highway's influence.

Also along this 9-mile stretch are four "bike bus stops." You're invited to hitch up your bike to the back of the bus and ride back to town. If you ride the 9 miles from Coronado to Imperial Beach and don't want to ride back—no problem. At the path's end, at Palm Avenue in Imperial Beach, you'll find a bike bus stop. And if you're taking the bike-and-pedestrian ferry home from Coronado to San

Diego, it's still no problem: A bike bus stop lets you off only a few blocks from the ferry.

Food Facilities Nearby: Many, many cafes along this route.

Restrooms: Tidelands Park; Glorietta Bay Park; Silver Strand State Beach and Nature Preserve.

Special Precautions: Watch for sun and heat exposure. Definitely wear a hat on this ride and bring plenty of water. Lock your bike. This area has many bike thefts.

Best Parking Lot: Ferry Landing Marketplace; Silver Strand State Beach.

Directions: To Ferry Landing Marketplace from Interstate 5, take the Coronado exit, Highway 75. Go over the bridge. It becomes 3rd Street in Coronado. Go about a quarter-mile. Turn right onto B Avenue. Cross 2nd Street and 1st Street. The entrance to Ferry Landing is on 1st and B.

For More Information: Visitors' Information Center, 1111 Orange Avenue, Coronado, California 92118. Tel.: (619) 437-8788 or (800) 622-8300.

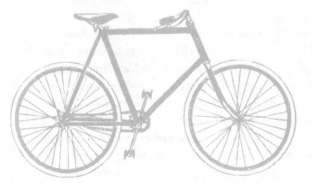

2. The Ojai Valley Trail

General Description:

This 9.5-mile "must-ride" trail, called "the most sophisticated of California's rail trails," won the 1989 Cal-Trans Award for excellence in transportation facilities.

Level of Difficulty: Easy.

Type of Scenery: Everything from urban to golf course to Christmas-tree farms.

Condition of Pavement: Excellent.

General Background:

In the late 1960s with the demise of the Ojai citrus orchards, the Southern Pacific Railroad was forced to abandon the spur between the city of Ojai and Ventura. The Ventura/Ojai spur went unused until 1981, when the county of Ventura bought the right-of-way to build a trail for the equestrians, cyclists, joggers, and walkers clamoring for trails in this increasingly urbanized area. The county, which depends almost exclusively on user fees to finance its public recreation areas, came up with a distinctive solution to funding this trail: utility companies lease the right-or-way *underneath* the trail, paying upwards of $40,000 a year. This provides more than enough money to pay for the upkeep of this trail.

The Bike Path:

When you ride on this fairly flat trail, you're riding a state-of-the-art creation. A 10-foot-wide asphalt path for bikes parallels a 10-foot-wide wood-chip path for horses. To further separate the two groups, there's an attractive 4-foot-high post-and-rail fence. If there are conflicts on this trail between the two groups, we haven't heard about them.

Highway 33 runs up the valley from Highway 101. It is *the* way to get to the city of Ojai from the coast and has become a very busy, traffic-congested road. The path parallels this highway, but is often separated enough to give a sense of isolation from the noise and fumes. You shouldn't expect a rural ride here, but you will be riding through plenty of pretty land, past Christmas-tree farms and orchards, through several park areas and golf courses.

The trail begins at Foster Park in Casitas Springs and ends near Soule Park and Golf Course. You'll cross several major roads along the way. Our favorite sight here was a horse and rider standing at a crosswalk. The Walk/Don't Walk light was triggered by an equestrian-level push button.

Food Facilities Nearby: Delis and shops along the way.

Restrooms: Foster Park; Oak View Community Park; Libbey Park.

Special Precautions: None.

Best Parking Lot: Foster Park.

Directions: From Highway 101, take the Highway 33 exit. Go north. Take the Casitas off-ramp and make a complete loop. Follow signs to Foster Park.

For More Information: The County of Ventura General Services Agency, Recreational Services, 800 South Victoria Avenue, Ventura, California 93009. Tel.: (805) 654-3951.

3. The Embarcadero and Mission Bay Park

General Description:

The Embarcadero, Mission Bay Park and the Bay Shore Bikeway make up a complex system of bike paths and bike lanes throughout the city of San Diego and the county.

Level of Difficulty: Easy to average.

Type of Scenery: Shoreline, flood-control channels, and very urban areas.

Condition of Pavement: This system is expected to be under construction through the end of the decade.

General Background:

The city of San Diego and San Diego County have many miles of bike paths, but they tend to be rather fragmented. While these paths are terrific aids to cyclists trying to get around the city, they aren't especially suited to family recreational cycling.

However, the county is currently completing the Bay Shore Bikeway, a bikeway of more than 20 miles that's a composite of bike paths and on-street bike lanes running north from Imperial Beach. Much of that ride will be on-street and only for experienced cyclists who are comfortable in traffic.

For family cyclists, we suggest in the city of San Diego the several miles of paths around Mission Bay Park, with both bike paths and wide sidewalks. Expect crowds. You may also ride on Fiesta Island (in the middle of Mission Bay), on bike lanes alongside usually slow-moving traffic.

The Embarcadero, also popular for cycling, is quite crowded. It runs for about 3 miles from San Diego's downtown area to Spanish Landing.

This bike system is in flux. Expected soon is a 4-mile path leading from the Bay Shore Bikeway to Otay Lake. Another path will lead from the bikeway to the Sweetwater Reservoir, following the channelized banks of the Sweetwater River. County cycling facilities are undergoing massive construction right now; when they near completion, there should be some terrific rides.

You can get a free, complete, county-wide map of the bike paths and bike lanes by calling (619) 231-BIKE.

For Up-to-Date Construction Information: City of San Diego Bicycle Coordinator, 1010 Second Avenue, Suite 800, San Diego, California 92101. Tel.: (619) 533-3110.

The County of San Diego Bicycle Coordinator. Tel.: (619) 694-2811.

4. The Shoreline Trail and the Upper Rio Honda Trail

LOS ANGELES COUNTY, CALIFORNIA

General Description:

A series of connected trails totaling almost 30 miles, stretching from Long Beach Harbor, North Long Beach, Hollydale, Bell Gardens, Montebello, and Rosemead, and gradually climbing in elevation to end near the mountains.

Level of Difficulty: Average.

Type of Scenery: The harbor and shore; very industrialized; Interstate 710; Whittier Narrows Dam; Peck Park.

Condition of Pavement: The county is beginning to repave many of these trails.

General Background:

More than 90 miles of paved paths stretch through Los Angeles County. Two of those paths are quite lengthy central arteries—this path and the San Gabriel River Trail (see separate entry). The two paths run somewhat parallel to each other. By creating bikeways that went to the mountains and to the beach, planning officials hoped to allow families access to recreational facilities without needing to use the family car.

These paths represent a tremendous commitment to cycling as a transportation option. The Lario Trail required the agreement of 13 separate municipalities, as well as their commitment to carry out the decisions made on the county level.

The Bike Path:

This path consists of four individual trails, all of which are connected: the Shoreline Trail, about 4 miles of path along San Pedro Bay, operated by the city of Long Beach; the Lario Trail, extending from the Shoreline Trail toward the mountains; the Los Angeles River Trail, a 4.5-mile trail branching northwest from the Lario Trail; and the Upper Rio Honda Trail, a continuation of the Lario Trail, so named because it follows that river. The ride currently ends near El Monte.

The first section of this ride, the Shoreline Trail, is flat and quite crowded. This boardwalk-style path is open to cyclists, but don't expect to get up much speed, unless you are up with the dawn and out riding. Even then, you'll have to contend with people.

Ride east along the path from Shoreline Park. You'll ultimately reach Alamitos Bay and Alamitos Bay Beach. This is the end of the line for this bike path, but adventurous cyclists can ride on-street for about a mile, crossing the bay on an automobile bridge. Continuing down Westminster Avenue, you can pick up the San Gabriel River Trail (see separate entry) on the east side of Alamitos Bay.

If you don't want to chance the bridge (you share a lane with traffic) ride back to Shoreline Park. Just west of the park, the Shoreline Trail connects to the Lario Trail.

This trail heads north along the channelized Los Angeles River. You'll be paralleling I-710 for about the next 10 miles, riding through the city's industrial centers. At John Anson Ford Park, the path crosses the river on a bike bridge.

Heading toward the mountains there will be a very gradual elevation increase. When the bike path crosses the Imperial Highway, look for the Los Angeles River Trail branching to the left. This trail continues to follow I-710, and ends in Maywood at Atlantic Boulevard.

The main trail follows a northeasterly direction. You'll come to Whittier Narrows Dam, a major recreation area where you can again connect to the San Gabriel River Trail. This flood-control dam is operated by the U.S. Army Corps of Engineers and offers outdoor activities, a nature center, and a visitor center. To reach this area, you'll have a short but quite steep climb up the dam face.

North of the recreation area, the trail changes names. It is now called the Upper Rio Honda Trail, since you are now following that river rather than the Los Angeles River. This last section of about 8 miles is relatively flat. It leads to Peck Water Conservation Park, a reservoir which allows recreational fishing and picnicking.

For the Family Cyclist: If you are interested in a short, family-oriented ride and don't want to bother with the beach scene, you might consider the Whittier Narrows Dam. This is the point of convergence for several different trails—the Lario Trail, the Upper Rio Hondo Trail, and the San Gabriel Trail. In addition, the small path around the reservoir adds a bit of scenic waterway for youngsters. If you have some cyclists in your group who want a short ride and others who want to explore, this recreation area makes a good home base. Don't let children ride alone here, though, and don't ride here near dusk. We are sorry to say that there have been some serious incidents along some sections of this trail.

Food Facilities Nearby: Snacks available along the Shoreline Trail.

Restrooms: Shoreline Park; John Anson Ford Park; Grant Rea Park; Whittier Narrows Dam; Peck Park.

Special Precautions: Ride with a friend. This trail runs through some areas where harassment of cyclists is occasionally a problem.

Don't ride along these trails at dusk.

Best Parking Lot: Shoreline Park; Whittier Narrows Dam.

Directions: To Shoreline Park: Take Interstate 710 south all the way to San Pedro Bay. Before you get to the piers, turn onto Ocean Boulevard. Look for the park on your right.

To Whittier Narrows Dam: At the intersections of Highway 60 and Highway 19, look for signs to the recreation area. It's nestled into the corner made by the two highways.

For More Information: Los Angeles County Bike Map Hotline: (213) 244-6539.

The County of Los Angeles Department of Parks and Recreation, 433 South Vermont Avenue, Los Angeles, California 90020. Tel.: (213) 738-2961.

5. The San Gabriel River Trail

LOS ANGELES COUNTY, CALIFORNIA

General Description:

A 38-mile ride with some spectacular views of the city and the ocean.

Level of Difficulty: Average.

Type of Scenery: Whittier Narrows Dam; some native landscaping; a somewhat natural river channel; several other dams and some birding sites.

Condition of Pavement: Repaving is in process.

The Bike Path:

Parts of this trail are spectacular, with flowing water and lots of vegetation, but you will be riding through some isolated areas. Don't ride alone.

This trail follows the San Gabriel River as it tumbles out of the San Gabriel Canyon. It begins at the L.A. National Forest Ranger Station on Highway 39, in the San Gabriel foothills, and runs to the east end of Long Beach's Alamitos Bay. The trail passes through many municipalities, including Azusa, Irwindale, Baldwin Park, El Monte, Pico Rivera, Santa Fe Springs, and Bellflower. Unlike other rivers in the region, this river remains in a semi-natural state. Flood control depends on an extensive system of reservoirs and dams, so you'll frequently ride near water.

Riding south from the ranger station, you'll come to

the Santa Fe Dam, 5 miles from the start of the ride. Most of these first 5 miles run through rather isolated areas. About 10 miles from the Santa Fe Dam is Whittier Narrows Dam, an important recreation area with connections to several other bike trails, including the Lario Trail and the Upper Rio Honda Trail (see separate entry). There is also a path around the reservoir.

The rest of the ride runs near Interstate 605, passing the Long Beach Pistol Range, Eldorado Nature Center, and Eldorado Park to end at San Pedro Bay. Just before the bay, you can leave the trail, turn left onto Westminster Avenue, and ride west on an automobile bridge (you must share a lane with traffic). On the bay's east side you can pick up the Shoreline Trail (see separate entry) and the Lario Trail.

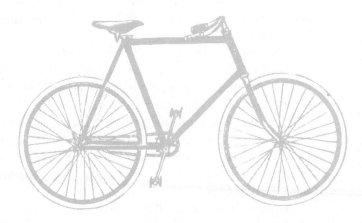

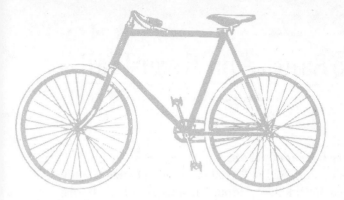

Food Facilities Nearby: None.

Restrooms: Santa Fe Dam; Whittier Narrows Dam.

Special Precautions: Do not ride these trails alone. Do not ride at dusk. Ride with a friend or, better yet, with a group.

Best Parking Lot: Whittier Narrows Dam; Santa Fe Dam.

Directions: To Whittier Narrows Dam: At the intersection of Highway 60 and Highway 19, look for signs to the recreation area. It's nestled into the corner made by the two highways.

To Santa Fe Dam: From Interstate 210, take the Highway 39 exit south. Turn right immediately onto Gladstone Street. This will take you to the recreation area.

For More Information: The County of Los Angeles Bike Map Hotline: (213) 244-6539.

The County of Los Angeles Department of Parks and Recreation, 433 South Vermont Avenue, Los Angeles, California 90020. Tel.: (213) 738-2961.

6. The Santa Ana River Trail

General Description:

An existing trail of 26 miles through Orange County, with planned additions through Riverside and San Bernadino Counties that will create a 75-mile-long trail.

Level of Difficulty: Average.
Type of Scenery: Seashore, urban areas, reservoirs, mountains.
Condition of Pavement: Repaving is ongoing.

General Background:

This is a trail in transition, with many changes being made. County authorities and the Army Corps of Engineers are building one of the nation's longest bike paths—75 miles—which will extend from the mouth of the Santa Ana River through the cities of Santa Ana and Anaheim to end in the foothills of the San Bernadino Mountains.

Twenty-six miles of the path, through Orange County, currently run along the channelized Santa Ana River. The Corps of Engineers is repaving this section, adding native landscaping and building new parks. The route through Riverside and San Bernadino Counties is in the planning stage.

The Bike Path:

This 26-mile path takes you up a gentle 2 percent gradient from the mouth of the Santa Ana River to the mountains. Near the seashore, you'll ride the levee system and will cross the river on several bike-and-pedestrian bridges.

There are several small parks along the river here. The first is Talbert Wilderness Preserve, an area with a developed portion of about 5 acres accessible only by bike path, with restrooms and water fountains and an interesting display of native coastal plants. In Santa Ana, you'll come to Centennial Regional Park, on the east side of Edinger Avenue and the river trail, with drinking fountains, restrooms, and picnic tables.

Throughout this very urban segment of the path, the river is channelized with concrete. After 17th Avenue, the river is channelized with stone riprap and is slightly more attractive. Edna Park, north of 17th Street, is a small park with drinking water. Next comes Anaheim Stadium and an area known as "the pond," the location of an ice hockey rink.

At Katella Avenue in Anaheim, you must cross the river on an automobile bridge with a 10-foot-wide bike lane. North of this bridge is a small, informal park area where you may see some horses from the nearby stables. Then the river turns sharply south. You'll cross the river at Imperial Highway and at Gypsum Canyon Road on bridges similar to the Katella Avenue bridge.

Then you'll enter a more natural area and come to two parks. Yorba Regional Park is a very large county-operated park. Swimming is forbidden, as in all Orange County parks. Featherly Park, also called Canyon View RV Park, is privately operated.

Here the stone riprap disappears from the riverbanks, and the river becomes prettier. Currently, the trail ends at the Green River Golf Course. The path becomes a roadway, Green River Drive.

The Corps of Engineers intends to landscape some parts of this ride quite soon. Other segments may not be completed until 1998 or later, but most should be replanted before the end of the decade. The plans emphasize xeriscape landscaping techniques similar to those used so successfully in Tucson's Rillito River Park Bike Path (see separate entry).

Food Facilities Nearby: At several urban centers along the ride there are sandwich shops and small restaurants.

Restrooms: At most parks along this route.

Special Precautions: Ride with a friend. This is an urban area.

In the afternoons, expect strong headwinds from the ocean.

Best Parking Lot: Huntington Beach State Park; Centennial Regional Park; Yorba Park.

Directions: To Huntington Beach, from Highway 1, the Pacific Coast Highway, take the Brookhurst Street exit. Turn south and head directly into the park. The mouth of the Santa Ana River, where the bike path begins, is at the southerly end of the parking lot.

To Centennial Regional Park, from Interstate 405, travel east on Edinger Avenue to Fairview. The park entrance will be near this intersection.

To Yorba Park, take Highway 91. Take the Imperial Highway exit. At La Palma, turn east. After 2 miles, you'll see the entrance to the park on the south side of the road.

For More Information: Riverside County Regional Parks and Open Space District, P.O. Box 3507, Riverside, California 92519-3507. Tel.: (909) 275-4310.

County of Orange Bikeway Coordinator, 300 North Flower Street, Santa Ana, California 29702. Tel.: (714) 834-3137.

For Orange County Bike Maps: (714) 834-3111.

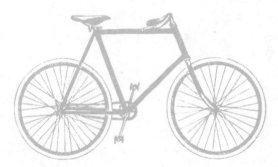

 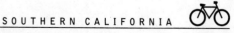

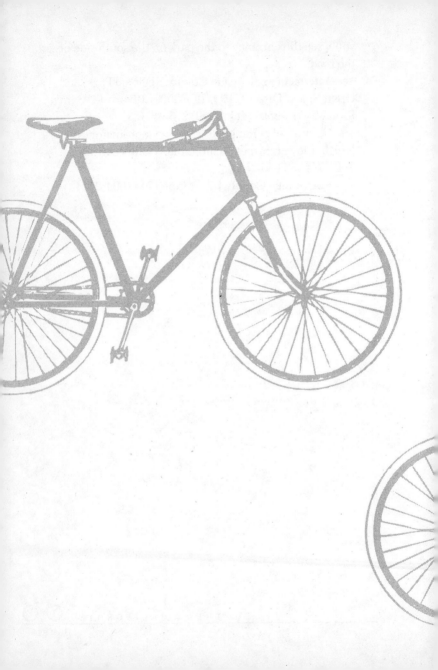

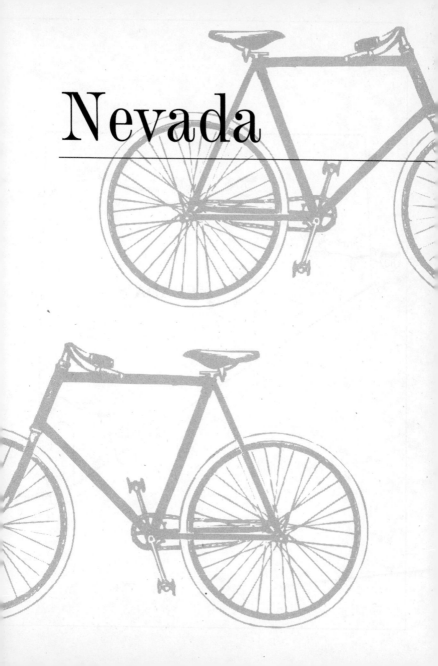

Nevada

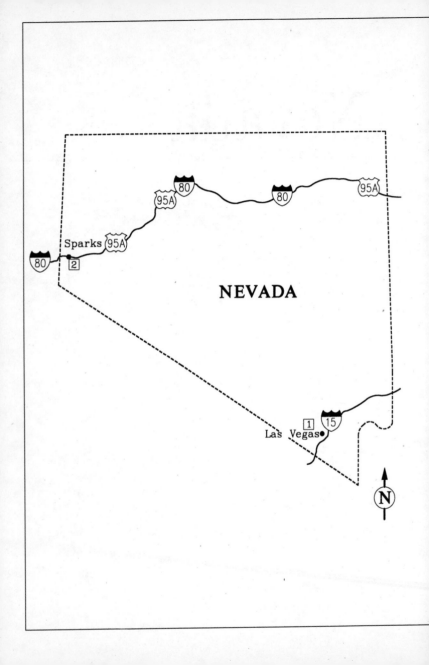

Nevada

1. Red Rock Canyon National Conservation Area

LAS VEGAS, NEVADA

General Description:

A 14.7-mile ride through protected federal land on a one-way loop road shared with cars, with very steep grades for the first 5 miles followed by a 1,000-foot descent.

Level of Difficulty: Very challenging!

Type of Scenery: The Keystone Thrust Fault; steep sandstone escarpments; plants and animals of the Mojave Desert, including numerous herds of wild burros.

Condition of Pavement: This is a one-way *on-road* ride!

General Background:

The federal Bureau of Land Management recently designated this a "conservation area," equivalent (almost) in protective status to a "national park." Red Rock Canyon, the seventh BLM area to receive this designation, needed the extra help. In 1995, more than 1 million people visited this delicate desert area.

Red Rock Canyon is suffering environmental stresses similar to those suffered by Utah's Zion Canyon (see separate entry). Red Rock staff are watching the shuttle-bus experiment in Zion closely. If Zion thrives, the BLM *may* close Red Rock to motor traffic and Red Rock visitors may have to take a shuttle, walk, or bike through the canyon.

The Bike Path:

We suggest you ride here *very* early in the morning. The loop road opens at 7 A.M.—the best time for cyclists. This is a two-lane, one-way road. The speed limit is 35 miles per hour, and there are no large trucks. Cyclists *should* have plenty of room to ride safely, but after 10 A.M. you'll contend with car fumes and honking horns.

A word of warning: The "one-way" designation applies to bicycles as well as cars. If you decide the elevations are too steep, you *may not* turn around and ride back down. You must continue your ride or *walk* your bike back. Cyclists riding downhill at high speeds against the traffic flow have caused serious accidents.

You'll begin from the visitor center by climbing more than 1,000 feet in 5 miles. But take heart. After that climb, it's downhill all the way back. As you climb, you'll find plenty of places to stop and rest. Calico Vista and Sandstone Quarry have great views and terrific photo possibilities. When you get to the next scenic area, White Rock, you're at the top.

As you being your descent, you'll find some switchbacks that require careful attention. Watch out also for loose gravel and falling rocks. Box Canyon and Pine Creek Canyon are good rest stops with hiking trails.

At 12.6 miles from the visitor center, you leave the canyon and ride a state highway, 159, to return to the visitor center. Be cautious: you'll be riding a highway with lots of two-way, high-speed traffic for the next 2 miles. If you have youngsters or cyclists who dislike highway traffic, you may choose to arrange a vehicle pickup at this point.

For the Avid Cyclist: There are several dirt roads in this conservation area where cycling is permitted.

Food Facilities Nearby: Light snacks at the visitor center.

Restrooms: The visitor center; Sandstone Quarry; Willow Spring; Pine Creek Canyon.

Special Precautions: This ride, requiring considerable skill and physical fitness, is not a ride for young children or for novice cyclists.

The loop road is *one-way*. BLM officials are serious about this. Cyclists must finish the loop. You may not ride against traffic.

The only drinking water available is at the visitor center. *The Mojave Desert gets hot.* The canyon frequently reaches 105 degrees. Bring lots of water.

Bring sunscreen and a head covering.

Watch for snakes in the rocks.

Best Parking Lot: Red Rock Canyon Visitor Center.

Directions: From I-15, take Nevada Highway 159 west about 15 miles. You'll first enter the conservation area boundary. About 7 miles into the area, you'll find signs for the visitor center and the scenic loop drive, on your right.

For More Information: The Bureau of Land Management, Las Vegas District Office, P.O. Box 26569, Las Vegas, Nevada 89126. Tel.: (702) 363-1921.

2. The Truckee River Bicycle Path

General Description:

A 6.2-mile path following the Truckee River as it flows through the cities of Reno and Sparks.

Level of Difficulty: Average.

Type of Scenery: Ten separate city parks nestled into the bends of the Truckee River; excellent bird-watching sites; thickets of willow, alder, wild rose; large stands of mature cottonwood.

Condition of Pavement: Good.

General Background:

The Truckee River begins in California at Lake Tahoe (see separate entry), flows out of the mountains and through the foothills of the Sierra Nevadas, then crosses a desert to empty into Pyramid Lake in northwestern Nevada. It's a trip of about 75 miles.

When John Charles Frémont first saw the river in 1844, he was impressed with the its powerful flow and crystal-clear water. Frémont loved the river's unusual cut-throat trout, which he called "salmon trout." In their honor, he named the river "the Great Salmon River." The name didn't stick. Eventually the river came to be called the Truckee, after an important Paiute leader.

Today, the water in the river is nothing like the water Frémont saw. The river is in considerable need of protection. Everyone has a claim to the Truckee's water—farmers, industrialists, housing developers. During the late summer and early fall, much of the Truckee is bone-dry. The river used to be an important migratory rest stop for a wide variety of birdlife, but unless the people who grab the water change their attitudes, this river's days are definitely numbered.

The Bike Path:

Sparks, Reno, and Washoe County have set up a system of interpretive parks along the water's edge similar to the system along the American River Parkway (see separate entry).

The path's eastern beginning is at East Greg Street in Sparks. You'll ride first through some industrial areas, then enter Cottonwood Park, the farthest east of the river's chain of 10 public parks. Until you reach the park, the ride is hot and sunny. But as soon as you reach Cottonwood Park, you'll find shade under the huge old trees. From here, much of the path will be shaded by these friendly trees.

Between Cottonwood and Glendale, the next park on the path, the cottonwood trees become so thick that you'll lose sight of the river from time to time. The feeling of isolation, of being hidden in a forest, is a welcome respite in this region's open landscape. You may also see willows, alder, wild rose, currant, and chokecherry along these banks.

Several of the parks along this chain have been designated "watchable wildlife" areas. If you're lucky, you may see raccoon, muskrat, deer, or even beaver. The path currently ends near the western boundary of Reno, although another 10 miles may be added on through Washoe County within the next few years.

Food Facilities Nearby: None.

Restrooms: At all public parks along the bike path from April until the snow flies in November.

Special Precautions: None.

Best Parking Lot: The beginning of the path in Sparks at Greg Street; Cottonwood Park, the easternmost public park on the path.

Directions: To get to the beginning of the path at Greg Street in Sparks, from I-80 take the McCarren Boulevard exit and head south. After several blocks, turn left onto Greg Street. Pass Franklin Street. The river and path will be on your right. Look for signs marking the start of the path.

To get to Cottonwood Park, from I-80 take the McCarren Boulevard exit and head south. After several blocks, turn left onto Greg Street and then right onto Spice Island. Cottonwood Park is at the end of the road on the riverbank.

For More Information: Sparks Leisure Services Department, 98 East Richards Way, Sparks, Nevada 89431. Tel.: (702) 353-2376.

Washoe County Parks, tel.: (702) 785-6133.

Reno City Parks, tel.: (702) 334-2270.

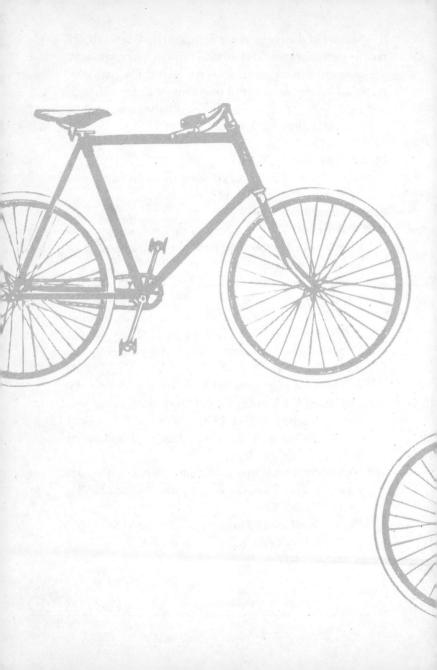

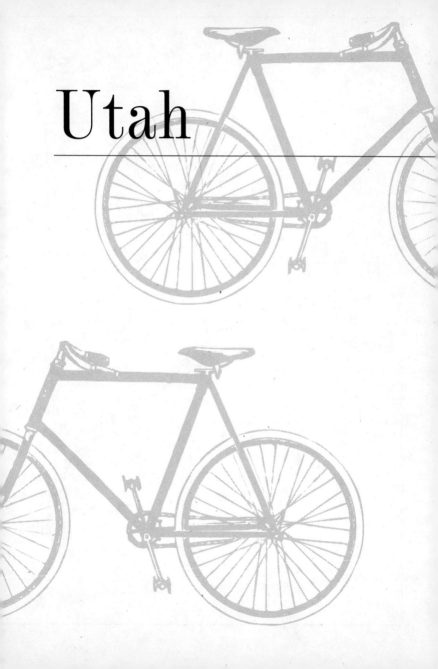

Utah

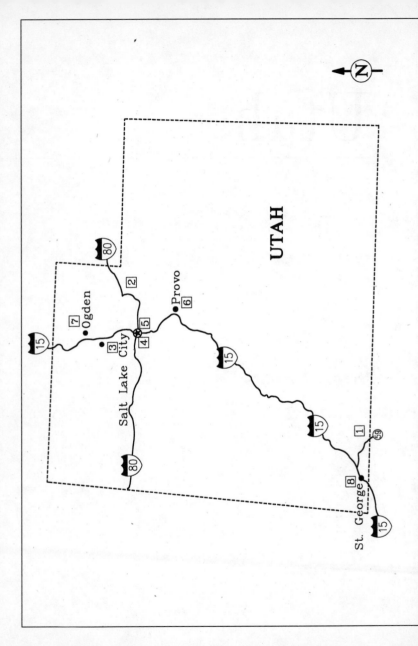

Utah

1. Zion National Park Bike Path and Zion Canyon

General Description:

A 2-mile path that winds through Virgin River wetlands, connecting with the 7-mile road through Zion Canyon, open only to bikes, pedestrians, and shuttles, beginning in 1997.

Level of Difficulty: First 2-mile section: average. Canyon road: challenging.

Type of Scenery: Along the bike path: the oasis-like world of the Virgin River; the desert ecology of the canyon slopes rising above the river; 4 steel bridges crossing the river.

Along the canyon road: Watchman Mountain; the Court of the Patriarchs; the Emerald Pools; Weeping Rock; the Temple of Sinawava; the Narrows.

Condition of Pavement: Excellent.

General Background:

Zion Canyon is smothering. After a heavy day of tourism, the plants and the animals can't breathe. Lead, cadmium, and other heavy metals are strangling them. The canyon's high walls trap the motor emissions, which fall to the ground and asphyxiate the delicate plants.

And then there's the noise. Much of the canyon's beauty lies in its spirituality and solitude. But when the 7-mile road is bumper-to-bumper and each diesel tourist bus brings 105 decibels of noise echoing off the canyon walls, you can forget meditating on God, life, and soul. All you want is a pair of earplugs and a quick escape route.

The invasion of motor vehicles has been relentless. In 1993, 2.5 million visitors came to Zion Canyon and more than 4,000 tour buses lumbered up the narrow road. But take heart. Their days are numbered.

Beginning in 1997, private motor vehicles will no longer clog Zion Canyon Scenic Drive. Park-operated shuttle buses, fueled by propane to decrease air and noise pollution, will carry visitors from site to site. For the first time in decades, you'll be able to visit Zion Canyon and share the peace and natural majesty experienced by the Anasazi, the Paiute, and the Mormon people.

The road *will* be open to cyclists and walkers. The ride, when the cars and noise and fumes are gone, promises to be one of the most beautiful bike rides in the world.

The Bike Path:

The 2-mile bike path opened in 1995 as the first stage of the conversion project. Gaining about 200 feet in elevation along its 2-mile length, the path begins at the park's Watchman campground under the 6,500-foot-high Watchman Mountain.

The path heads north along the Virgin River to intersect the Zion/Mt. Carmel Highway and the Zion Canyon Scenic Drive. (The Zion/Mt. Carmel Highway will remain open to traffic; it is the Zion Canyon Scenic Road which will close in 1997.)

Novice cyclists and families with young children will love this bike path. It crosses the Virgin River four times on gently arched steel bridges with 10-foot-wide wooden decks. The views from the bridges are spectacular—and surprising. In the midst of this seemingly unrelenting desert environment, you'll ride through a plush world vibrant with vegetation.

Graceful Fremont cottonwoods, with their gently bending trunks and their soft green leaves, dominate the scene, but there are also box elders, hardwoods belonging to the maple family. Annuals and perennials cover the river's banks. You may see mule deer, porcupine, ducks, geese, bald eagles, and maybe even a great blue heron.

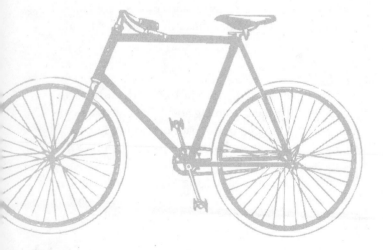

Above the canyon floor on the canyon walls is a totally different ecosystem of piñon and juniper trees, "the Pigmy forests of the Southwest." These short and tubby trees, which survive on limited water, have heights of 6 or 7 feet but rotundities to compensate for their stuntedness.

As you leave the bike path and ride up the canyon road, the walls gradually close in above you, slowly eclipsing the sun and the sky. At the canyon's mouth the walls are a half-mile apart, but by the road's end there's just enough room for the river.

As you ride along the canyon's scenic road, you pass the mountains named by the religious men who passed by here: the Mountain of the Sun, the Three Patriarchs (Abraham, Isaac, and Jacob), Cathedral Mountain, and the Great White Throne. You pass Angels Landing and the Organ and the Pulpit.

Ultimately, you reach the final destination: the Temple of Sinawava, where the sheer walls tower overhead like the pillars of God's mansion. To continue past here, you must lock your bike and wade in the water. This is the region called the Narrows. Bring water-walking footgear. Bare feet are dangerous: The rocks are slippery and the current is strong.

Bring bike locks and plan on lots of short side trips. Along the 7-mile scenic road you'll find many foot trails that lead to sites like the Emerald Pools and Weeping Rock. You may also want to stop at Zion Lodge, about midway along the drive, to freshen up or eat. Just north of Zion Lodge is the Grotto, a pleasant picnic area.

The round-trip from the Watchman to the Narrows and back is about 18 miles.

 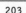

Special Note: The town of Springdale, also beleaguered by tourist traffic, dreams of building a bike path leading from Springdale's hotels into the park. No specific construction dates have been set to our knowledge, but if you're staying in Springdale you might ask about this.

Food Facilities Nearby: Zion Lodge; Springdale.

Restrooms: The visitor center; the campgrounds; Zion Lodge; Grotto Picnic area; at the trailheads for Weeping Rock, the Temple of Sinawava, and Canyon Overlook.

Special Precautions: Elevation differences mean climatological differences. Dress accordingly.

Bring plenty of water. Temperatures reach 105 degrees.

Bring hats and sunscreen.

Rattlesnakes are evenly distributed throughout the canyon.

Bikes *may not* leave the pavement. If cyclists fail to respect park vegetation, bikes will be banished along with the cars.

Smoking is not permitted on the bike path.

Best Parking Lot: The Zion Canyon Visitor Center; the Watchman trailhead; when the canyon road is closed, park officials hope cyclists will park in Springdale and ride their bikes to the canyon.

Directions: Utah State Route 9 runs through the park and the town of Springdale.

For More Information: Zion National Park, Springdale, Utah 84767-1099. Tel.: (801) 772-3256.

2. The Historic Union Pacific Rail Trail State Park

PARK CITY TO ECHO RESERVOIR, UTAH

General Description:

A 27-mile rail trail following the course of Silver Creek and the Weber River to Echo Reservoir, mostly through natural areas and farmlands.

Level of Difficulty: Average.

Type of Scenery: The banks of Silver Creek and the Weber River; Echo Reservoir and, by the end of the decade, the Jordanelle Reservoir; wetlands and meadows filled with birdlife like sandhill cranes, bald eagles, and great blue herons; some semi-urban areas; for a short while, biking within the I-80 right-of-way.

Condition of Pavement: Asphalt paving, begun in 1995, will continue over several years in this recently opened state park. Until then, the ride will be rough but possible on hybrid and mountain bikes. The railroad ballast has been "bladed"—smoothed down—and ¾-inch gravel covers the bed. For up-to-date paving information, contact the agency below.

General Background:

In 1869, just as the Union Pacific Railroad was preparing to pound in the Silver Spike at Promontory Point, silver was discovered in the Wasatch Mountains at the southern edge of a mountain meadow. These two factors spurred a profound shift in the region's economy. People arrived and the mining industry thrived. The Union Pacific built a 27-mile broad-gauge line down from its cross-continental line to Park City, the region's silver-mining center. The Union Pacific held on to this line until 1989, when plans for the state corridor park began to take shape.

The Bike Path:

Children old enough to ride distances but not quite ready for backcountry riding will love this corridor park. There's a sense of adventure here—but you're never too far from safety and civilization.

The ride begins in Park City, once a rough mining town, now a ski-and-golf resort. This is Utah at its greenest. The path follows a creek and river through mountain-framed meadows and wetlands that are rest areas for migratory birds, including the hypnotizingly beautiful sandhill cranes.

As you ride the 7 miles from Park City to Star Pointe, look back over your shoulder at the receding Wasatch Mountains. After Star Pointe, still following the Silver Creek, the path runs between the eastbound and the westbound lanes of Interstate 80, then passes through Wanship, named after the leader of the Cumumbas, a band of intermarried Utes and Shoshones who lived here before the Europeans.

After Wanship, the path leaves the highway and you'll see beaver dams and cottonwood thickets. In the winter you may see bald eagles roosting on these branches, waiting for rainbow trout. The area is also a winter range for deer and elk.

Finally comes Echo Reservoir, open to the public for boating, swimming, and camping. The waters are silt-laden, with extensive mudflats at the southern end. About 80 million years ago, this region was rich delta land, the mouth of an immense river that once flowed out of the mountains to the west. The gravel and boulders brought by the river formed an alluvial fan which eventually hardened, forming the Echo Canyon Conglomerate—the steep walls that rise so spectacularly above the town.

Food Facilities Nearby: Park City, Wanship, and Coalville have restaurants. Otherwise, bring your own supplies.

Restrooms: At each parking/staging area.

Special Precautions: This state park, about 125 feet wide, is bordered by private land. State officials ask you to respect private property.

Bring your own water and basic emergency supplies.

Best Parking Lot: Park City, Coalville, or Echo Reservoir.

Directions: To the Park City parking area from Salt Lake City: Take exit 145 from I-80. Turn right onto Route 224. Turn left onto Kearns Boulevard (Route 248), right onto Bonanza Drive, and left onto Prospector Avenue. The parking lot is on your right, beyond the Park City Plaza.

To the Park City parking lot from U.S. 40: Take Exit 4 (Route 248) into Park City. Turn left onto Bonanza Drive and left onto Prospector Avenue. The parking lot is on the right past the Park City Plaza.

To the Coalville parking area: Take Exit 164 from I-80. Bear right off the ramp. Turn left onto Main Street, then left onto 200 North.

The Echo Reservoir parking area, the northernmost limit of the trail, is currently under development. For up-to-date information, check with the agencies listed below.

For More Information: Historic Union Pacific Rail Trail State Park, P.O. Box 309, Heber City, Utah 84032-0309. Tel.: (801) 645-8036.

Utah Division of Parks and Recreation, 1636 West North Temple, #116, Salt Lake City, Utah 84116-3156. Tel.: (801) 538-7221.

3. Antelope Island State Park

General Description:

A 7.2-mile bike lane along a causeway over Great Salt Lake; a short ride in traffic; a 3-mile loop trail along the northern shore of the largest island in the lake.

Level of Difficulty: Average.

Type of Scenery: Rugged mountains and green pastureland; a buffalo herd of 600 animals; the eerie waters of the Great Salt Lake; in the distance, expanses of water and pristine mountain ranges of stark beauty.

Condition of Pavement: As of 1995, the island loop is a single-track dirt trail that the state hopes to pave soon. The causeway is paved.

General Background:

Antelope Island is a geological anomaly. Some of the oldest rock in Utah pokes through the island's surface, so that 3-billion-year-old rocks sit beside 100-million-year-old rocks.

Yet the lake in which the island sits is one of the region's newest formations. The 2,000-square-mile lake is really just a meager puddle, a sad remnant of the glory days when the original lake, Lake Bonneville, spread across Utah. In its hey-day—15,000 years ago—Bonneville extended north into Idaho and south to what's now

Lund, near the Arizona border. Today's Provo and Salt Lake City would have been in the middle of that hundreds-of-miles-wide lake.

Evidence of the late, great Lake Bonneville remains today. You can see its former shoreline. Terraces that look like flat roads run high up along the surrounding mountain ranges.

Antelope Island, Great Salt Lake's largest island, is about 15 miles long, 5 miles wide at its widest point, and about 800 feet above the lake. Shoshone once lived here. The explorer John Charles Frémont saw the island in 1843. A few years later, the trapper Osborn Russell walked the land.

In the 1960s, the island's northern section became a state park, and by the 1980s the whole island was state owned. State development has been minimal, although a few improvements—a better swimming beach and a visitor center—are planned.

The 3-mile Buffalo Point trail may be paved by 1998.

The Bike Path:

This unique family ride has been open to the public only since 1994. There are three separate stages to this ride: the bike lane on the causeway, a short bit of on-street cycling, and the dirt loop around Buffalo Point.

To begin the ride, park your car at the gate to the park on the mainland and ride the 7-mile causeway over the lake. We should caution you: On this causeway ride, you'll be biking on a separate lane, but beside traffic that may be moving at 40 or 50 miles per hour. (If you want to avoid this, you may drive across the causeway and park there.)

As you ride over the water, you'll see rugged hills and mountains in every direction. If you look carefully, you should see the road-like terracing cut into the mountains from Lake Bonneville's ancient shoreline. Ahead, you'll have a full view of Antelope Island. To the north are the Promentory Mountains. In the distance are the snow-covered Hogup Mountains. On a particularly clear day you can sometimes see the Sierras. Behind you are the Wasatch Mountains, covered with snow from late fall to early spring, and the spectacular Wasatch Front.

You'll see a plethora of birdlife. Shore birds like seagulls, kerlews, and grebes make their home here, hundreds of miles inland from the Pacific. The Great Salt Lake sits in a major north-south migration corridor, so you're likely to see lots of migrating flocks.

The island itself is a haven for wildlife. The domestic stock has been replaced by a herd of about 600 American bison. This particular herd, with its unique gene pool, has played a major role in revitalizing other inbred herds across the continent. The island also hosts antelope, deer, elk, coyote, bobcat, and fox. Soon to be introduced: Rocky Mountain bighorn sheep.

When you reach the island and the end of the causeway, you'll have a short ride on a paved road that will run by the beach. This road is open to motor traffic.

Then you'll come to the 3-mile off-road loop around Buffalo Point. Until this loop is paved, you should have a fat-tired bike. This loop is easy enough for most children, but there will be several rocky areas where you should expect to walk your bikes. Officials expect to pave these rugged sections first. The loop connects to a dirt road that's quite suitable for novice cyclists and that leads back to the paved road.

For the Avid Cyclist: A paved road runs up to Buffalo Point, at an elevation of 4,785 feet above sea level. This is a steep climb; cyclists are welcomed. Also, a rugged backcountry single-track ride on this island, the White Rock Bay Loop, is available for experienced backcountry cyclists. Permits are required.

Food Facilities Nearby: A small store on the island.

Restrooms: At the visitor center on the island.

Special Precautions: The island's water supply is not dependable. Either bring your own water or check with the park service before you start out.

June and July are almost too hot for biking on this island. If possible, plan to go in late spring or in the fall.

Check with the state park service about opening and closing times. The park is just becoming operational and has yet to set a regular schedule.

Best Parking Lot: At the causeway's mainland end.

Directions: From I-15, take Exit 335 near Syracuse and Layton. There are signs for Antelope Island. Go west on Antelope Drive for about 7 miles, until you reach the causeway gate.

For More Information: Davis County Tourism, P.O. Box 305, Farmington, Utah 84025. Tel.: (801) 451-3286.

Antelope Island State Park entrance gate, tel.: (801) 773-2941.

4. City Creek Canyon Road

General Description:

A 5.5-mile ride through a wild canyon only a few minutes from downtown Salt Lake City.

Level of Difficulty: Challenging.

Type of Scenery: A flowing creek hemmed in by steep canyon walls; several picnic and barbecue areas; a city reservoir and water-filtration plant.

Condition of Pavement: Good.

General Background:

City Creek is an important water resource for Salt Lake City. The creek flows out of the Wasatch range, carving this canyon that remains semi-wild, right behind the state capitol building.

The canyon road once facilitated mining operations in the canyon, but those have long been closed down. Now the road mainly services the water-filtration plant.

The canyon road is currently shared by motorists and cyclists by way of an unusual system that seems to be quite successful. On "bicycle-only" days, the odd-numbered days of the month, cars are forbidden. Bikes are forbidden on even-numbered days and on holidays. Since this schedule is obviously subject to change, we suggest you check ahead for confirmation.

The Bike Path:

Begin your ride at Memory Grove Park, a park established in memory of the veterans of World War II. The road will rise gently for the first several miles, and you'll enjoy lush vegetation along the creek banks.

About halfway up the canyon, the climbs become steeper. The last mile or so is quite steep, with an elevation change of more than 500 feet.

At the top, you'll come down to Rotary Park, a good place to picnic before riding back down. Be cautious when descending since cyclists are not the only people who use this road; it is open every day to pedestrians and to water-district vehicles. City officials ask that cyclists limit their speeds down the canyon road and also obey the keep-to-the-right rule, especially when rounding canyon bends.

Food Facilities Nearby: None.

Restrooms: At Memory Grove Park.

Special Precautions: Limit speeds during descents! Other people—including pedestrians—use this road.

Best Parking Lot: Memory Grove Park.

Directions: Take the 600 North exit from Interstate 15. Go east. Turn right onto 300 West. Go south. Turn left on North Temple Street. Pass Main Street and State Street. Turn left onto B Street, and look for Memory Grove Park.

For More Information: Julie Eldredge, Salt Lake City Transportation Division, 333 South 200 East Street, Salt Lake City, Utah 84111. Tel.: (801) 535-6630.

5. The Jordan River Parkway

General Description:

A 4.5-mile path that follows the banks of the Jordan River through the downtown area of this state capital.

Level of Difficulty: Easy.
Type of Scenery: A highly developed city bike path located near the confluence of Interstates 80 and 15.
Condition of Pavement: Good.

The Bike Path:

Plans are for the bike path to parallel the length of the Jordan River, from Utah Lake to the Great Salt Lake. This path is currently in the process of being developed. It may be necessary to bike on-street for some of the 4.5 miles.

When development is complete, the city expects to have a fully developed urban park and bikeway, complete with playgrounds, canoe launches, and a wheelchair exercise course.

Long-range plans call for the bikeway to connect with other bikeways built along the river. Since construction is ongoing, it may be best to check on the progress with the agency listed below.

Food Facilities Nearby: None.
Restrooms: Riverside Park and Cottonwood Park.

Special Precautions: None.

Best Parking Lot: The Utah State Fairgrounds.

Directions: From Interstate 15, take the 600 North exit. Head west on 600 North Street. Turn south onto 900 West Street. Turn right onto North Temple Street. The Utah State Fairgrounds are near North Temple and 10th West Streets.

For More Information: Julie Eldredge, Salt Lake City Transportation Division, 333 South 200 East Street, Salt Lake City, Utah 84111. Tel.: (801) 535-6630.

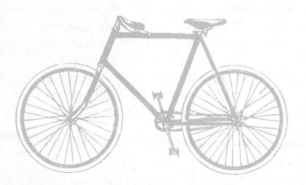

6. The Provo River Parkway

General Description:

A 16-mile path following the Provo River from Utah Lake State Park through the city and up Provo Canyon.

Level of Difficulty: Average, then challenging: a gentle climb from the lake through the city; a 6 percent grade up the canyon.

Type of Scenery: Utah Lake; the riverbanks under the shade of birch and willow trees; the steep walls of Provo Canyon; Bridal Veil Falls and an aerial tramway rising to a restaurant above the falls.

Condition of Pavement: About 40 percent asphalt-covered; the rest covered with slag, a solid foundation suitable for all bikes, but rougher than asphalt. More sections will be paved soon.

General Background:

The Provo River tumbles down out of the Uinta Mountains and empties into Utah Lake. The water from Utah Lake flows into the Jordan River, then on into the Great Salt Lake—130 miles of contiguous riverbanks and lakeshore.

Once upon a time, the state envisioned a bike-and-recreation parkway joining the various parks, to be called the Provo–Jordan River Parkway. The state even created a "parkway authority" back in the 1970s to implement the plan.

Today, few people know the plan exists. The "authority" no longer exists, but the Provo River Parkway stands as proof of how beautiful—and popular—such a parkway would be. These 16 miles drew 1 million visitors last year. A few energetic trail enthusiasts continue to lobby for completion of the parkway. We hope their voices will be heard.

The Bike Path:

Although this path parallels the four-lane U.S. Route 189 that climbs the canyon, path designers tried to keep the recreation trail distanced from the highway whenever possible. A 100-foot vegetation buffer separates the highway and the river; the path tends to hug the fast-flowing water, which helps block out the traffic noise.

The path begins at Utah Lake State Park and Boat Harbor, at the west end of Center Street. It heads east, meandering through a wetland area with good bird-watching opportunities. Several stops along the way provide interpretive information.

Next the path crosses Interstate 15 and heads north. This is the most urban segment of the ride, but the river and landscaping help by creating a sense of a more natural setting. The path links four major urban parks: Wilderness Park, Riverside Park, Exchange Park, and Ron Last Park.

Leaving the city and entering the canyon, you'll ride below towering mountains, beneath the canyon walls. Nearby is the 11,500-foot Mt. Timpanogos. You'll begin a steady climb up a 6 percent grade, passing several scenic viewing areas, picnic tables, and hiking trails. There are several hiking trails that leave from the viewing areas.

The last of the canyon parks, Bridal Veil Falls, is also the end of the bike path. The waterfall is spectacular—a 600-foot drop—and the aerial tramway is equally spectacular. With a distance between terminals of 1,753 feet, local tourism groups claim their tramway is "the steepest in the world." The tramway goes up to the top of the falls, where there's a restaurant.

Food Facilities Nearby: The restaurant at Bridal Veil Falls.

Restrooms: At each public park, from spring through fall.

Special Precautions: None.

Best Parking Lot: Bridal Veil Falls; Geneva Street; Utah Lake State Park and Boat Harbor.

Directions: To Bridal Veil Falls from I-15, take the Utah State Highway 52 exit (also called 800 North) in Orem. Go east. Bear northeast on Route 189. Bridal Veil Falls is about 5 miles up the canyon.

To Geneva Street, take the Provo West Center Street exit. Travel west. Turn right onto Geneva Road. Go 4 blocks. Cross the river. Parking area and trailhead are on the left.

For the state park, take Center Street to the lakeshore.

For More Information: The Provo City Parks and Recreation Department, Box 1849, Provo, Utah 84603. Tel.: (801) 379-6600.

The Utah County Travel Council, Historic County Courthouse, 51 South University Avenue, Suite 111, Provo, Utah 84601. Tel.: (801) 370-8393 or 1-800-222-

7. The Ogden River Parkway

General Description:

A 3.1-mile path following the Ogden River through the city.

Level of Difficulty: Easy.

Type of Scenery: The mouth of Ogden Canyon; the George Eccles Dinosaur Park for children; the Utah State University's botanical gardens.

Condition of Pavement: Good.

The Bike Path:

The Ogden River, known for its tremendous trout fishing, tumbles out of the massive Wasatch Mountains through Ogden Canyon on its way to Great Salt Lake. The city of Ogden sits at the mouth of Ogden Canyon at the base of the mountains.

City officials are protecting the south bank of the river by building a system of publicly and privately financed parks. The bike path is integrated into the preservation plan. The ride is esthetically lovely, with only two major road crossings despite the urban environment.

This path is meant to be a family recreation path. In keeping with the intention, it begins at Dinosaur Park, an educational attraction for children, with about 60 exhibits.

Following the riverbank, the path touches on botanical gardens and an arboretum. It then goes under a highway by way of a special bike tunnel and ends at Washington Boulevard in the city center.

Officials hope to extend the path another 5 or even 10 miles to the west. There are also long-term dreams of connecting with the Historic Union Pacific Rail Trail (see separate entry).

Food Facilities Nearby: Cafe at Dinosaur Park.
Restrooms: Dinosaur Park; Big D Park; MTC Park.
Special Precautions: Speed limit of 15 miles per hour.
Best Parking Lot: Dinosaur Park.
Directions: From I-15, to Dinosaur Park, take Exit 12. Travel east on 12th Street to the mouth of Ogden Canyon. There will be signs to Dinosaur Park. Turn right onto Valley Drive, and right onto Park Boulevard.
For More Information: Ogden City Parks and Community Services, 1875 Monroe Boulevard, Ogden, Utah 84401. Tel.: (801) 629-8284.

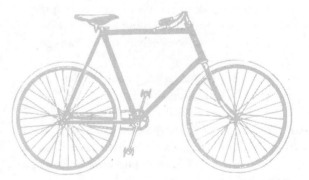

 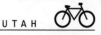

8. The Virgin River Bikeway

General Description:

A flat path of a bit more than 4 miles that runs through the golf-resort town of St. George, along the Virgin River, and up a protected tributary, the Santa Clara River.

Level of Difficulty: Very easy.
Type of Scenery: A bird-watcher's paradise along the banks of the river; urban and suburban through the town.
Condition of Pavement: Excellent.

General Background:

The city of St. George, in the state's southwest corner, is nicknamed "Utah's Dixie." When the rest of the state is covered with snow, the St. George area is warm and sunny with near-perfect temperatures for outdoor activities. Biking is a particularly popular winter activity for St. George snowbirds.

The existing nugget of paved bike path is just the beginning of a hoped-for 30-mile spiderweb system that may materialize by decade's end. It's a visionary plan: The trail, currently running along the river's north side, will also follow the south bank. There will be 5 river crossings. The trail will tie in with Snow Canyon State Park and surrounding communities.

222

The Bike Path:

For now, you'll have a ride of 4 miles. One segment follows the north side of the Virgin River for about 2 miles. It then leaves the riverbank and, paralleling Hilton Drive, heads into the historic center of St. George.

There is also a 2-mile segment of path along the south side of the Virgin River. You can bike across the river at the Man-O-War Bridge, also a bridge for vehicular traffic.

The path traversing the north riverbank begins in the southern part of St. George at the Man-O-War Bridge and runs to the confluence of the Virgin and Santa Clara Rivers. The path's Hilton Drive staging area is adjacent to the Southgate Golf Course. The St. George Tabernacle, the second tabernacle built by the Mormons, is visible straight ahead. You'll also get a view of the famous red-rock cliffs surrounding St. George, as well as the "black ridges," the large plateaus settled by Brigham Young's people.

Food Facilities Nearby: In St. George, numerous sandwich restaurants and inexpensive cafes.

Restrooms: At both staging areas.

Special Precautions: This is desert country; be careful of the heat and bring plenty of water.

Best Parking Lot: The Man-O-War parking area.

Directions: From Interstate 15, take the Hilton Drive exit and follow the signs.

For More Information: The St. George Leisure Services Department, 175 East 200 North, St. George, Utah 84770. Tel.: (801) 634-5869.

If you have information about a bike path

that ought to be included in this series, please contact:

Wendy Williams

P.O. Box 14

Mashpee, Massachusetts 02649

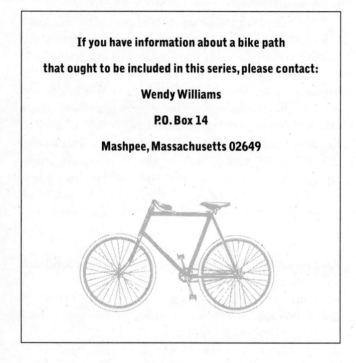